Do-It-Yourself Herbal Treatments

How to Cure Common Ailments Using the Power of Nature

By: Bonnie Smith

9781681275215

PUBLISHERS NOTES

Disclaimer – Speedy Publishing LLC

This publication is intended to provide helpful and informative material. It is not intended to diagnose, treat, cure, or prevent any health problem or condition, nor is intended to replace the advice of a physician. No action should be taken solely on the contents of this book. Always consult your physician or qualified health-care professional on any matters regarding your health and before adopting any suggestions in this book or drawing inferences from it.

The author and publisher specifically disclaim all responsibility for any liability, loss or risk, personal or otherwise, which is incurred as a consequence, directly or indirectly, from the use or application of any contents of this book.

Any and all product names referenced within this book are the trademarks of their respective owners. None of these owners have sponsored, authorized, endorsed, or approved this book.

Always read all information provided by the manufacturers' product labels before using their products. The author and publisher are not responsible for claims made by manufacturers.

This book was originally printed before 2014. This is an adapted reprint by Speedy Publishing LLC with newly updated content designed to help readers with much more accurate and timely information and data.

Speedy Publishing LLC

40 E Main Street, Newark, Delaware, 19711

Contact Us: 1-888-248-4521

Website: http://www.speedypublishing.co

REPRINTED Paperback Edition: 9781681275215:

Manufactured in the United States of America

DEDICATION

This book is dedicated to Marc. Thank you for the inspiration.

TABLE OF CONTENTS

CHAPTER 1- THE UGLY TRUTH BEHIND PRESCRIBED MEDICATIONS

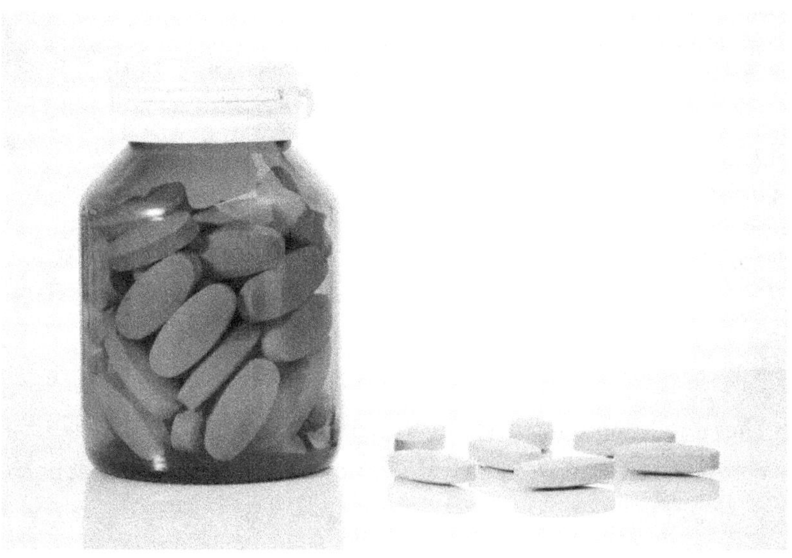

According to the American Medical Association Journal, over 100,000 Americans die in hospitals every year due to side effects from regularly prescribed medications. Throughout America, a huge amount of medication is prescribed on a daily basis. The medical community openly acknowledges that fact that it does not have any cure for several common diseases that affect people. Most allopathic medicines have side effects that can range from mild to severe.

The reason for this is that most of these chemicals have certain toxic properties. This is why there have been so many prescription drugs that got pulled from the market after enjoying several years of FDA approval. The sad thing is that very few doctors nowadays bother to inform patients about possible side effects due to close and cozy relationships with the pharmaceutical industries.

Half of the truth is that pharmaceutical companies will only tell doctors as much as they want to and not reveal the complete picture. Therefore, the doctors are not completely to blame because they cannot warn patients against side effects of chemicals they are not aware of.

The trouble is that the business is so profitable is that these medicine manufacturers are more concerned with profits and FDA approval rather than the overall effect on the patients. This is one reason why several doctors are now beginning to recommend complementary alternative treatments, like herbal therapies and medicines.

Here are some interesting facts:

• The totally amount of annual profits made by pharmaceutical companies through sale of drugs in the United States alone is over $100 billion

• More than 25% of all prescription drugs available contain plant derivatives More than 80,000 types of plants are used all over the world for medicinal purposes

• Over 75% of the global population depends on herbal remedies for regular treatment There are several choices available for people who are looking for alternative remedies, including Acupuncture, Yoga, Qigong, Tai chi, Ayurveda, hydrotherapy, massage therapy, homeopathy, energy medicines, holistic approaches, and aromatherapy. In fact, the number of herbal remedies available for different ailments equals (if not exceeds) the number of regular drug treatments provided by pharmaceutical companies. The point is that prevention always was and always will be better than any cure, mainstream or alternative.

The advantage of herbal remedies is that they move an individual towards a lifestyle more geared toward prevention and cure in the early stages of any affliction. Pharmaceutical drugs work only after the problem has development, they do not try to prevent problems because then the manufacturing companies would go into a loss. This is where herbal remedies leave the mainstream drugs behind. This is also the reason why so many people are daily turning to herbal therapies. Herbal remedies treat the cause of the disease and not the symptoms (like conventional drugs). Herbal remedies also have almost no side effects.

Chapter 2- Benefits of Alternative Cure

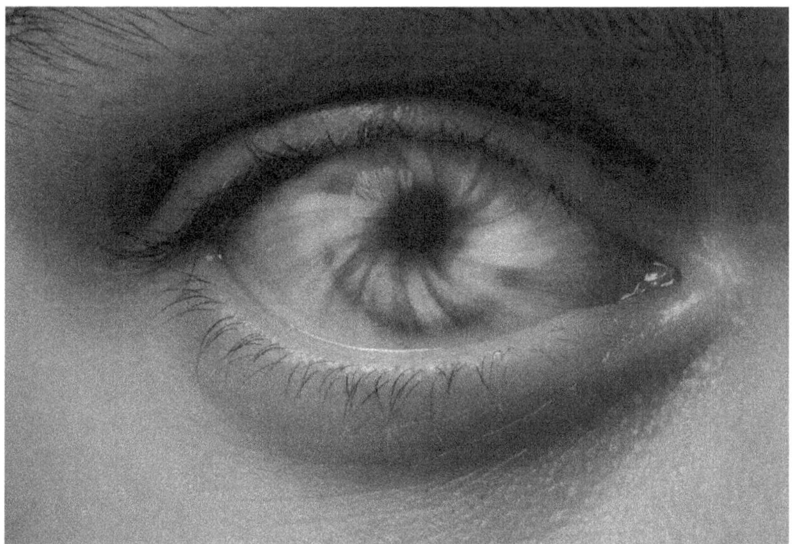

Alternative medicine believes that natural health is a consequence of a variety of different sources coming together. Thus it chooses the best from various options available, in order to provide good health. It does so by building the strong points, preventing the weak ones, and generally dictating a lifestyle that is naturally healthy.

Alternative medicine branches that promote natural good health include herbalism, natural hygiene, naturotherapy, and nutripathy. Nowadays it has become common to provide these, as complementary therapies to conventional methods of treatment. Terms like alternative medicine and natural health always seem to get associated with the Far East. It should be noted that most of the core concepts behind natural health are of European origin. In the old age the only health care that was available to the common man was self-care. While medical science existed in a very rudimentary state, it was by no means as prolific as it is today.

Most of the "doctors" in that era were referred to as "folk healers" (people who heal other people) and their medical qualification was nothing more than a short apprenticeship under some sort of superior.

At the time of the Revolutionary War, practicing the art of medicinal healing was looked upon as a diversion, something to dabble in when you had time to spare. It was supposed to be something that an individual did when not doing a regular job. Folk remedies were handed down from one generation to the next. Men and women who had learned these remedies simply applied them to everyday life like their predecessors. In this way, matters like childbirth, injuries, and illness were taken care of.

Geographical distance and biological diversity naturally made these folk remedies different in different places. So, while the roots of such healing can be traced to Europe, once they had been adapted to the Americas, they were not so readily recognizable. In 1830, Frances Wright and other reformers and activists started the Popular Health Movement. This was a period when advances in medical science were forcing contemporary doctors to think in terms that would have been sacrilegious to their elders.

Frustrated by these new developments, proponents of the Popular Health Movement sought to enforce the usage of older methods into the practice of modern medical professionals. While some good has resulted (in the long run and with the help of understanding provided by modern research), it has to be admitted that the Popular Health Movement also caused some medical blunders. Some natural health concepts that arose as a result of the Popular Health Movement are: Hydrotherapy, Herbalism, Eclectic Medicine, and Natural Hygiene.

Thomsonianism is one of the earliest approaches to modern western herbalism and it was founded by Samuel Thompson around the year 1820. The Association of Eclectic Physicians, an organization of herbals doctors, was found in Wooster Beech. At its very height, eclecticism was practiced by over twenty thousand qualified doctors in the United States. By 1939, medical schools were being largely influenced by philanthropists, and when these schools failed to support eclecticism, it slowly died out.

Hydrotherapy was another branch of natural health and it concerned itself with the application of water to the human body. Though using only water as means of staying healthy might sound a bit silly, for that time period it was a good thing.

Hydrotherapy advocates were very vocal about the importance of personal habits such as diet, dress, clean water, fresh air, exercise, sunshine, and herbs. Personal hygiene as it is followed today was not always such an important issue. Hydrotherapy was conveying a very important message.

Origins of hydrotherapy can be traced back to Europe in the Roman era when spas and hot mineral springs were a common way for people to cleanse their bodies. The European system of hydrotherapy was first introduced to the United States in 1844 by the founder of Natural Hygiene, Dr. Joel Shew. Dr. Shew later on enhanced hydrotherapy by focusing on its other aspects like fresh air, lots of sunshine, a good diet plan, and an exercise routine. In 1853 he established the college of Hygieo Therapy.

The American Natural Hygiene Society was founded in 1948. Eventually, hydrotherapy had to give way to allopathy. This was largely brought about by the fact that the people supporting allopathy viewed hydrotherapy as a science of quacks because hydrotherapy was so closely associated with the female social activists of that era.

The core belief of natural health therapy is that all issues related to health, sickness, and healing can be overcome through simple means like prevention and a change in individual lifestyle. Natural health follows the oldest rule of medicine: prevention is better than cure. In view of this, natural health therapies are supposed to be totally in control of the individual and not the doctor or healer.

The "natural" in the term natural health literally refers to the physical world in which we live, or nature. This is but another way of saying that according to natural health therapy all disease and illness is nothing more than a natural reaction to some other natural action.

It is important to remember that natural health does not have anything to do with faith or psychic healing which are supernatural concepts and hence, by definition, not part of nature. This difference is also the biggest distinguishing factor between natural health therapies of European origin and Eastern alternative medicinal theories that often rely on belief systems such as spirituality, karma, ancestral forces, personal auras, or energy flows. None of these can be perceived by our normal senses and hence the Europe-born natural health theories do not subscribe to them.

Going even further, natural health does not concern itself with the origin of life, any religious beliefs, extra-dimensional worlds, magic, and new age mysticism. All natural health says is that all health and sickness can be affected by simple natural therapies. At its most basic level it can be said that natural health therapy refers to only one thing: biological factors of health, especially as they apply to everyday life in western society.

Do-It-Yourself Herbal Treatments

In its early history, the natural health movement did show considerable interest in hydrotherapy and the relaxation it offered through the usage of spas, steam baths, and other water cures. The more modern additions to natural health that concern themselves with the body-mind connection and how that relates to stress and tension are influenced by eastern alternative medical theories.

Having said that, what natural health therapy finally implies is that the human body has complete capacity to heal itself from most forms of sickness (of course, a broken bone cannot be fixed by altering your lifestyle, it needs to be put in a cast), mostly through prevention. So as far as natural health thinking goes, all healing is basically self-healing and this is considered to be a basic property of all things alive.

Vitalism

It is to be observed that as early 400 B.C., Hippocrates (who is considered to be the father of medicine) had written that, "The natural healing force within us is the greatest force in getting well". This is known as vitalism, also known as 'vis medicatrix naturae' (the inherent wisdom of the body). To put it simply, whenever there is something wrong with the body the doctor will attempt something, for example: using antibiotics to kill the infection perform surgery to remove a poisoned part or for amputation, put a broken bone into a cast, suture a flesh wound. All of these are part of the healing trade.

The catch is that the body of patient has to actively respond to all this treatment otherwise it is wasted. Vitalism makes the body to want to heal and get well. This is a well-documented fact that people who deal with their physical problems confidently and cheerfully heal faster than others. The precise reason as to why this happens is not understood but the fact is still undeniable.

Bonnie Smith
Holism

One explanation comes from the concept of Holism which says that the process of healing is a combined effort by the entire organism and cannot be achieved by any isolated part of that organism. The Holism concept can be traced to the time of Paracelsus, 1439-1541, who is credited with being the father of modern medicine. When Paracelsus treated patients he refused to pay attention to only that part which was showing symptoms of disease. Instead, he tried to treat the whole body as one whole entity.

Holism is not a symptom=cure sort of healing technique. It involves a careful study of the defensive abilities of each individual patient's body. Practitioners have to have the knowledge to differentiate between disease symptoms and the defensive or recovery systems.

What Holism believes is that when someone falls sick, their whole body has undergone some kind of weakness and has lost the balance of its strength. So the solution is to simply restore the strength of the body. All western natural health therapies rely on biological factors and the better developed psychosocial approaches are a modern addition.

Individualism

This concept is different in the sense that it places all responsibility for sickness and good health on every individual in a society. So everyone is responsible for their personal health. Individualism results from an awareness of the importance of individuals in a community and the resulting virtues of self-reliance and personal independence. Well-rounded individuals are both self-reliant and independent.

Victim-blaming

What this means is that if someone gets sick then the victim of the sickness did something wrong. While it might sound a little weird what it honestly means is that personal health is a personal responsibility and no one can blame someone or something else for his or her illness. It focuses on the self. Improve yourself because the environment around you is too big to change for one individual. In other words, health problems should be self-corrected and the obvious solution is a change in the victim's lifestyle.

Prevention

This is probably the most difficult concept for the modern day individual to grasp. Though everyone is aware of the phrase 'prevention is better than cure' there are few people who actually go the extent of preventing even the most obvious trouble (think about smoking, alcohol, high cholesterol foods, sugar, etc.). Prevention does not merely suggest that troublesome activities should be avoided. What is says is that improving health is better than fighting disease. It suggests the application of this to short term as well as long term negative effects. In the short term, a healthy body can easily ward off minor illnesses (like common cold) and injuries (razor cuts, skin peeling during sports activities for instance).

In the long term prevention suggests caution in all that is done today so that it does not result in adverse outcomes in the future. In other words, it too suggests a change in lifestyle for a healthier tomorrow. Reasonably good health can be achieved by everyone. What is even better that the means to do so do not have to acquire from anyone, the capacity to do so lies within us.

Chapter 3- Everything You Need to Know About Natural Herb Remedy

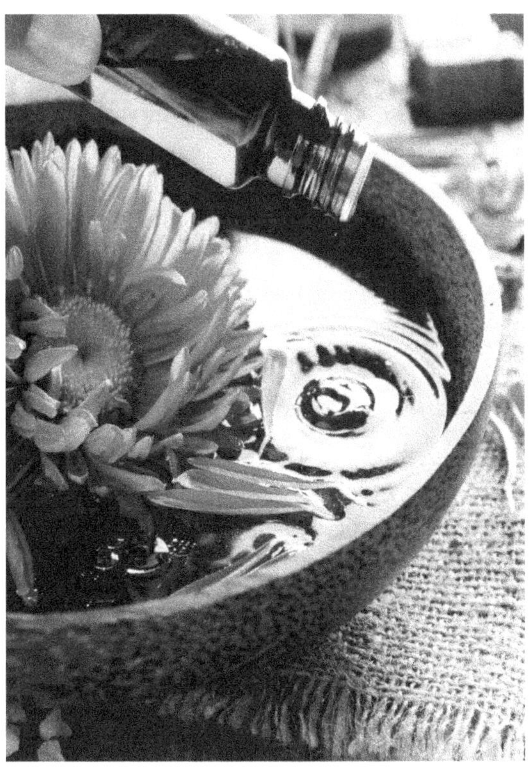

Any plant grown for culinary, medicinal and even spiritual value is called an herb. It is common practice that, from an herb plant only the green and leafy parts are used. The culinary usages are obviously different from the medicinal uses; in fact, it is often the case that the properties of culinary and medicinal herbs are entirely different to be found in the same plant. For example, medicinal herbs usually tend to be shrubs or woody plants.

Culinary herbs, on the other hand, are typically more leafy and soft. Interestingly, the seeds, berries, bark, root, or other parts of an herbal plant make great spices. These plants also bear edible fruits or vegetables. Culinary herbs are different from other vegetables in the sense that they are not the primary objects to be cooked or consumed. Instead, they are used to provide flavor when used as spices.

Botanical Definitions

Botanical science defines an herb as a plant that does not produce a woody stem. It usually dies in temperate climates. Death can be complete in case of annual herbs or the herb can simply go back to its roots in case of perennial herbs. Examples of herbs include: bulbs, peonies, hosta, grasses, and banana. The botanical term herbaceous means a plant having the characteristic of an herb or being leaf-like in color and texture. Herbalism

Herbalism is also known as phytotherapy. It is a very old folk medicine that is based on the use of plants and plant extracts. Human beings have been looking for healing powers in the vegetable kingdom for a long time. There are innumerable types of indigenous plants that have been used by people for centuries in the treatment of many ailments. The history of such usage is long and well documented.

Evidence has been found that sixty thousand years ago the Neanderthals living in present day Iraq used plants as medicines. Radiocarbon dating of the Lascaux caves in France has revealed that cave paintings dated between 13000-25000 BCE displays the use of plants as healing agents.

It must be appreciated that our forefathers spent several centuries slowly building upon the knowledge of their own predecessors to arrive at proper medical conclusions. It took many generations of trial and error to expand this knowledge base. The individuals who took upon themselves the task of following this line of reasoning and medical discovery are whom we today remember as "healers" or "Shaman".

An interesting aspect of plants is their seemingly infinite ability to synthesize aromatic substances like phenols and tannins. Plants also evolve alkaloids that serve as defense mechanisms against predatory microorganisms, insects, and herbivores. Plants and chemicals have a strong and historical relationship going back to several hundred millions of years.

The chemical interactions in a plant's metabolism, offense, and defense procedures are very complex. Human beings have found that many herbs and species that are used in seasoning of good often yielded useful medical compounds. In recent years plants have once again come into the foreground as the search for new drugs and dietary supplements have led researchers back into the plant kingdom.

Pharmacologists, microbiologists, botanists, and natural product chemists are literally going through the entire roster of plant species with a fine toothed comb looking for phytochemicals that could lead to the development of cures for several types of diseases. Already there are many drugs on the market that have been derived from plants.

Herbal treatment of diseases is nearly universal in all non-industrialized societies. Since they do not have the resources to set up pharmaceutical industries and are quite likely to be too impoverished to purchase modern day drugs, it should not be surprising that they rely on plants that they can grow to fight off illness.

In western society, the use of herbal medicine can be contributed to the accumulation of several traditions over a long stretch of time, finally culminating at the end of the twentieth century. Some of these influences are based on ancient Greek and Rome, the Ayurvedic principles from India, and Chinese herbal medicines. Some very common plant based pharmaceuticals that have been used by western physicians include opium, aspirin, digitalis, and quinine.

Background

In any living organism, chemical reactions define the metabolism rate and control normal metabolic activities. Some of these chemicals are known as primary metabolites (sugar and fat) and are found in nearly all plants.

Chemicals known as secondary metabolites are found in a limited number of plants. The functions of secondary metabolites can be very different. They could be used to produce alkaloids (poisons) for defense or to attract insects to enhance pollination. Most of the therapeutic chemicals derived from plants as well plant based modern drugs rely on the secondary metabolite chemicals in plants. A few examples are: inulin (roots of the plant dahlias), quinine (from cinchona), morphine and codeine (from poppy), and digoxin (from foxglove).

The National Center for Complementary and Alternative Medicine has started to fund clinical trials to improve the medical world's understanding of herbal medicine. Popularity In May 2004, the National Center for Complementary and Alternative Medicine conducted a survey. The focus of this survey was on people who had used Complementary and Alternative Medicines (CAM), what particular types of treatments were used, and why did the people choose for the complementary medicine option.

The results of this survey indicated that, with the exclusion of prayer, herbal therapy (or the use of natural products besides vitamins and minerals) was the highest used complementary and alternative medicine. 18.9% opted for herbal therapy over all other forms of complementary and alternative medicines.

Here are a few samples of medicines used in herbal therapy.

- A variety of plants (including artichoke) help to reduce the total serum cholesterol levels.

- Plants like black cohosh (and others that contain phytoestrogens or active estrogen) have proven effective in treating symptoms of menopause

- A limited number of studies have reported that the average length of common cold can be reduced by using Echinacea extracts.

- Garlic is an herb that provides multiple benefits like lowering of cholesterol levels, lowering blood pressures, and reducing platelet aggregation.

- Another highly diverse medicinal plant is black cumin (nigella sativa). Common ailments that can be cured using black cumin include: cough, pulmonary infections, asthma, influenza, allergy, hypertension, and stomachache. The seeds of black cumin are classified as carminative, stimulant, diuretic, and galactogogue. Seed powder or oil from black cumin can be applied externally in case of skin eruptions. Digestive tract problems including irritable bowel syndrome and nausea can be relieved by drinking peppermint tea.

- Rauvolfa serpentina is one of the oldest and most widely used herbs in India. It is applied for treating problems like insomnia, anxiety, and hypertension. This herb is also the foundation for the first plant based allopathic drug that was developed to combat high blood pressure.

- In some clinical trials it has been discovered that St. John's Wort, a most dangerous chemical, can be highly effective in cases of mild to moderate depression

- Another plant root that can be used in the treatment of sleeplessness is valerian.

Dangers of Herbal Treatments

All modern pharmaceutical drugs need to be prescribed due to dangers of side effects or allergic reactions, or possibly reaction with other drugs. This has resulted in the development of a myth about natural products, including herbalism, which has spread far and wide. The myth goes that natural products are safe. Or, anyone can take them without consulting an expert and they will do no harm. In the end, whatever we extract from plants, spices of curative agents, we are dealing with chemicals.

Over centuries the defense system of plants has led them to produce some very lethal chemicals. There are innocent looking plants that can give an adult nausea if a single leaf is smelled close closely. A small nibble of the same leaf by an infant can be fatal. Fortunately, most such plants are found deep in the forests where predators other than man are a threat.

Still, there are milder forms of toxins in plants much closer to us and even these can be lethal if caution is found lacking. For example, hemlock and nightshade are two plants that can prove to be fatal through carelessness. Also to be remembered is the fact that plants or herbal remedies are as likely to cause side effects and allergic reactions as other pharmaceutical drugs. However, these problems usually result from improper dosage and impurities.

Another danger is taking herbal remedies with conventional drugs when both perform the same task. In that case the cumulative effect will surely result in an overdose.

Is Herbal Treatment Effective?

Scientific studies provide indisputable evidence that the herbals extracts from plants can not only cure but also prevent certain types of diseases. Further evidence of the benefits of herbal medicine can be found in the fact that there are many modern pharmaceutical drugs available that use plant extracts. The need for caution comes in when reading the advertisements and other marketing materials for alternative medicines, even if they are plant based, 100% natural and completely safe.

There are no products on the market that will advertise boldly that they might not be effective in some cases. That sort of statement is usually hidden in the small print. That should not be criteria when choosing an alternative medication. There are cases where scientific studies have shown that people receive none of the medical benefits that the product claims to deliver. There are many alternative medicines on the market that have not undergone any sort of testing whatsoever.

The importance of scientific testing becomes apparent when you consider that these old-age natural therapy concepts were developed when there were no scientific controls and no test procedures. If someone wanted to try out a new herb, the easiest way is to try it on them first. Secondly, the human mind was not as well understood as it is today. For example, modern controls can easily make out the difference between a placebo effect, the body's ability to heal itself through its immune system, and the actual practical benefits of herbs. Without this understanding any herb, whether beneficial or not, can be made to look like a life saver.

Scientific investigation also helps to reveal the precise nature and structure of the chemicals in an herb. Which chemicals do what? How to they react with blood and other internal organs. What chemical combines where to produce what compound – finally resulting in a cure or relief? These are important facets of scientific testing that were not available in the days when herbal traditions were being established.

Most knowledge in those days was anecdotal and based on personal experience. Humanity and especially the medical workers know better today. It is always prudent to choose a medical treatment that has been proven safe and effective. It is possible for people to get so influenced by the natural healing movement that they will abandon conventional medicine altogether.

Avoid falling into this trap. Herbal therapies have just begun to be studied scientifically and until proven safe and sound should only be used as complementary alternative medicines, not the main treatment. The chemical composition of a lot of herbs is still not known so there is always the standing danger of violent reaction to an alkaloid. Do not underestimate this.

Standards Used in Different Countries

Different countries allot different legal status to different herbal ingredients. For example, Ayurveda, the alternative medicine therapy from India believes that heavy metals are therapeutic. The United States however believes that high levels of heavy metals are actually unsafe for normal consumption.

So Ayurvedic medicines are not granted the same status as regular drugs and they are certainly not FDA approved. Like other non-FDA-approved health products, Ayurvedic drugs are sold in the United States as dietary supplements and not medicines. This is merely an evasion because as per American laws, supplements do not need to be tested for safety or effectiveness.

In some cases even quality control of the active ingredients can be inadequate.

Usage

If you intend to use herbal remedies then it is always advisable to first have a detailed and frank discussion with your doctor. Keep in mind that herbal remedies can cause adverse reactions just like conventional drugs.

This risk is augmented when herbal remedies are taken in combination with prescription or over the counter drugs. For example, if you are taking medication for hypertension (these medicines lower blood pressure) and at the same time you take an herbal supplement with the same affect, there is a very high risk possibility of blood pressure dropping dangerously. There are also many supplements available that might contain herbs, which are to be strictly avoided during pregnancy.

Chapter 4- Herbology: A Chinese Method of Healing

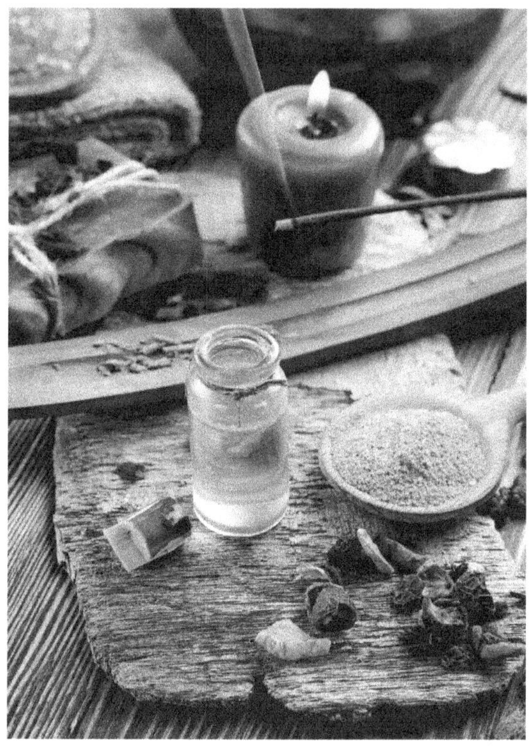

Herbology is the name given to the Chinese method of combining medicinal herbs. In this technique, which is one of the most widely used in Traditional Chinese Medicine (TCM), every herbal medicine is actually a cocktail of several herbs that are customized to individual patients. The doctor will assess the yin/yang condition of a patient in addition to studying the symptoms of the ailment.

The preparation of the medicine begins with the use of or two main herbs that target the ailment. The other herbs are added in order to adjust the yin/yang condition. Other ingredients can be added to cancel out toxicity or side effects resulting from the main herbs. This sort of herbal mixing to arrive at a formula that is suitable to individual needs is not easy.

A lot of experience and tutelage is required before a practicing of traditional Chinese medicine can perform the mixing independently. An important difference between traditional Chinese medicine and modern drugs is that the balance and chemical interaction of the ingredients a formula is considered more important than the individual ingredients.

Another quirk in Chinese herbology is that while it may be called herbology it will use all parts of a plant including: leaf, stem, flower, and root. In fact, some remedies will also use ingredients derived from animals and minerals. This has caused quite a bit of controversy because sometimes traditional Chinese medicine can call for ingredient from animals that are declared as endangered species (seahorses, rhinoceros, tigers, etc.).

Shennong is usually considered to be the first Chinese herbalist. It is said that Shennong tasted hundreds of herbs and experimented with them before passing on his knowledge of medicinal and poisonous plants to the farmers of China. He also wrote the first Chinese manual on pharmacology: the Shennong Bencao Jing. This manual lists approximately 365 medicines out of which 252 are herbal.

The manual is dated around the 1st century Han dynasty. One of the most important of such documents that were written by several master practitioners of Chinese herbology is the Bencao Gangmu. It was put together by Li Shizhen during the Ming dynasty. The contents of Bencao Gangmu are so potent that even today they are used for consultation and reference. Classification of Chinese herbs is in itself a very intricate process. Very broadly speaking, Chinese herbs are classified using methods such as those described below.

The Four Natures

The four natures are basically the yin and yang states and how effective an herbal medication is in bringing them into balance. Yin and yang degrees can range from cold (extreme yin), cool, neutral (warm), or hot (extreme yang). Before selecting herbs the doctor will make a careful study of the yin/yang balance in a patient. So if the patient has "internal cold" then an herb that has a "hot" yang value will be used and so on.

The Five Tastes

Some herbs are identified by their taste. While the taste in itself has no medicinal value in the absence of a better yardstick Chinese medicine associates the taste associated with an herb to the final effect. These five tastes are pungent, sweet, sour, bitter, and salty. Each taste has its own function. Pungent herbs are used to increase sweating, vitalizing blood and a more balanced Qi. Sweet herbs are used to tone and harmonize body systems.

Other sweet herbs help in curing excessive dampness by way of diuresis. Sour taste is meant to be astringent. Bitter tasting herbs help the body get rid of excess heat, empty the bowels, and reduce dampness by causing dryness. Salty herbs can help to soften up hard masses.

The Meridians

Meridians do not have anything to do with the Earth's meridians or magnetism. What they refer to is the precise organ that the chemicals in an herb target. So menthol which is pungent and cool is associated with lungs and liver. This means that since lungs are the organs that protect the body from cold and influenza the use of

Bonnie Smith
menthol can help to get rid of coldness in the lungs and also resist heat toxins.

Chapter 5- Different Types of Herbal Medicine

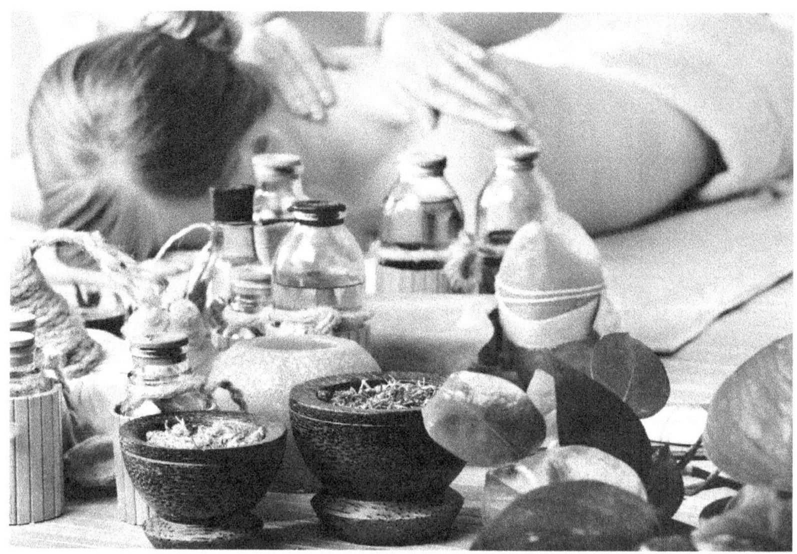

There are many positive aspects that herbal medicine has going for it. Unfortunately, the lack of adequate scientific understanding means that there is no way a doctor can completely take responsibility for what is being prescribed and hence the safety factor involved in taking herbal medicines is suspect.

The drugs that we normally take have to undergo thorough testing and need FDA approval. This entire process ensures that every single chemical in the medicine and its interaction with the human body (and resulting side effects) are well understood, documented, and scientifically demonstrable. While herbal medicines enjoy the reputation of being less complicated it should be remembered that they are manufactured by Mother Nature and she does not need FDA approval or scientific testing.

Fortunately, thousands of years of development have put herbal medicines into a certain safety zone that has helped many a human being with being cured. So herbal medicines might be risky but there is no need to worry if you take the simple precaution of consulting your doctor before consuming any herbal concoction.

Doctors are sort of walking pharmacopoeias and they know more about all those chemicals and stuff. They can advise you properly. Another thing to know with herbal medicine is that different cultures have resulted in different types of herbal therapies. Finally, thanks to the Internet and online marketing there is no shortage of frauds selling roots and leaves grown in their backyards.

Make certain that when you get herbal medicine it comes from genuine herbs. The wrong herbs might possibly contain toxic chemicals that make a trip to the hospital inevitable.

Some common forms of herbal medicines are as follows:

• You have probably come across the line "essence of ..." followed by some plant or flower when reading an ad for a cosmetic product. While Essences tend to get associated with cosmetic products due to massive advertising of those products, certain essential oils are always available for therapeutic purposes. The popularity of essential herbal oils processed through cold pressing or steam distillation is because many people prefer to get a massage than eating a pill. The most common benefit of essential oils is the help they provide in relaxing. They do not really cure any problems. Their major effect is to provide relief.

• Body massages can release toxins in the muscles, aiding relaxation.

• Head massages can likewise reduce heaviness or, in some cases, cure headaches. Similarly, chest massages using essence of certain herbs can help with congestion resulting from common cold.

- Pills or capsules. There was a time when this alternative was not available. It was a dark time for people who could not stand the taste of raw herbal medicines. The pills and capsules were a godsend for people who wanted to try herbal remedies but were unable to swallow. In order to convert an herb to pill form it first needs to be dried and crushed into powder. What is of interest is that there are hardly any herbal medicines available in pill or capsule form that target specific ailments. They act more like secondary medications to provide moral support to whatever primary medication is being taken. Professionals in herbal medicine believe that the drying and crushing of the herbs robs them of their potency. Others suggest that herbal medicine should be taken in its raw form for complete effectiveness. Anyway, if you are looking for specific herbal medicines instead of general health enhancers and supplements then this option is not for you.

- Infusions. The most popular form of herbal infusion is the drinking of various kinds of tea. Infusion involves the use of the delicate parts (leaves, seeds, and fruits) of an herbal plant and is quick to administer. Some ingredients of infusion tea could be stinging nettle, oat straw, red clover, raspberry leaf, and comfrey leaf. Infusions can be just the tea you drink normally (but using herbs instead of tealeaves) or what is known as Medicinal Strength Tea. Most herbal teas fall into this category though the preparation is slightly different. There are several recipes available on the Internet for making Medicinal Strength Tea.

- Poultice. For injuries, inflammations, cramps, or other spasmodic problems it can become necessary to apply the herbal mixture as a poultice. The required herbs are first macerated or chopped into small pieces. These are then applied directly to the affected area and covered with a hot and moist bandage. In some cases, the herbal mixture can be applied as a layer to the moist bandage before wrapping it around the affected area.

- Raw. As the name suggests, in this case the herbal medicine is taken in its most natural form without any additives or changes to make it palatable. Most people will run a mile in tight shoes to avoid this form of medication. It is the equivalent of taking a regular capsule, pulling it open, taking that powder, putting it on the tongue and trying to suck on it as if it were chocolate. Not done, well at least not if the taste buds are functioning normally. No wonder this method in unpopular. The good news is that most of the herbs that need to be taken raw can alternatively be soaked (or passed through) water to make medicinal strength teas, and those are much easier on sensitive palates. It is also believed that teas increase the effectiveness of raw herbs.

- Tinctures. There are very few kids who get exposed to this form of medicine these days but about twenty odd years ago no kid that got into a scrap in the field escaped the terror of tincture. These are basically herbal medicines in a liquid form. They can be for external as well as internal use. Modern incarnations are a lot milder that their older forms.

- Decoctions. A decoction is a liquid preparation made by boiling a medicinal plant with water usually in the proportion of 5 parts of the drug to 100 parts of water. Typically, certain specific parts of a plant like berries, roots, and herb-bark are used in this process. Depending on the consistency of the plant part being used, it can take up to two hours to prepare a decoction. This process extracts the flavor and increases the concentration of the herb through the process of boiling.

Do-It-Yourself Herbal Treatments

That more or less covers the different types of herbal medicines available. Depending on your requirement and personal taste you might need to take them in one of the above forms.

Chapter 6 - Herbal Diet Supplements: Hype or Truth?

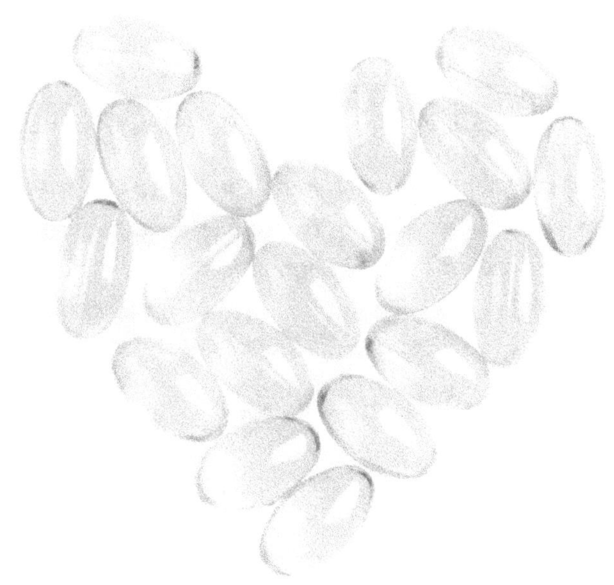

Herbal supplements are a type of dietary supplement that contain herbs. An herb (also known as a botanical) is a plant or plant part used for its scent, flavor, and therapeutic properties. Diet supplements derived from herbs usually contain more than one type of herb. The purpose of an herbal diet supplement is to increase the benefits that you get from your normal diet and to ward off the negative effects.

Herbal diet supplements are rich in vitamins, minerals, amino acids, etc. Obviously, dietary supplements are not meant to be used as treatments or cures of any disease or medical condition. They are more effective as preventative agents that help strengthen the body and the immune system to naturally ward off any infections or internal malfunctions.

For people who do not manage a balanced diet herbal diet supplements also supply necessary nutrients missing from regular diet. Many herbal dietary supplements can provide substantial aid for different types of medical conditions.

Some herbal diet supplements are:

- Ephedra. This supplement increases the body resistance towards common cold, helps in the treatment of asthma and upper respiratory problems. For people who work out regularly, ephedra is an important ingredient in most fat loss supplements.

- Magnesium. Minerals and salts are the biggest deficiencies in an unbalanced diet. Magnesium is essential in preventing kidney, thyroid, and heart disease. There are many herbal diet supplements rich in magnesium.

- St. John's Wort. Also known as Hypericum, Klamath weed, and goat weed, this supplement has been used for centuries in the treatment of mental disorders, nerve pain. In older times it was also used as a sedative and malaria cure. Nowadays, the common uses are treatment of depression, anxiety, and sleep disorders. It is typically consumed as a tea or in pill form.

- Vitamin E. Uncontrolled oxidation in our body can result in long-term damage. That is why our bodies generate antioxidants. However, if the production of anti-oxidants falls below safe levels then external supplements are required.

- One very potent anti-oxidant is vitamin E. Herbal diet supplements rich in vitamin E make good anti-oxidants.

- Copper. While metals and minerals are essential to the normal functioning of our body, sometimes they can fail to get absorbed properly.

- Zinc is essential for our body and there is nothing better than a copper rich herbal diet supplement. These supplements increase the absorption of zinc. The result is better protection against heart disease, and healthier skin and hair color.

- Folate. From a certain viewpoint, folates are required more than anything else because they can affect us down to our DNA. Folates are required for the production and maintenance of new cells (especially during pregnancy and infancy). DNA replication cannot take place without folates. Folates also prevent cancer causing DNA changes. Folate deficiency affects the bone marrow where most new cells are produced. Folates are needed to make new red blood cells and prevent anemia. As you can see, any deficiency in folates can be devastating in the end. One of the earliest indications of folate deficiency is anemia. Herbal diet supplements that have folates as major ingredients are always good for you, even if you do not have any problem currently.

- Iron. In the human body, the metal iron is more pervasive than any other. It plays an important part in several vital functions. Iron carries oxygen to the lungs and muscles in the form of hemoglobin. It acts as a means of transport for electrons between cells. It is a catalyst for enzyme reactions in tissues. Iron deficiency most commonly occurs in children and pre-menopausal women. It can easily prove to be fatal if left unchecked. Herbal diet supplements rich in iron can help to prevent such a situation.

- Vitamin B6 and B12. Vitamin B6 (pyridoxine) deficiency can lead to anemia, depression, dermatitis, and high blood pressure.

Vitamin B12 (cyanocobalamin) deficiency can lead to anemia, memory loss, and cognitive decline. It is most likely to occur among elderly people. In extreme cases, it can even cause paralysis. It is widely used in the treatment of alcoholism, depression, diabetes, hair loss, and stress. Vegans are especially at risk of B12 deficiency because vitamin B12 naturally occurs only in meats. If you are a vegan, then an herbal dietary supplement with vitamins B6 and B12 is an absolute must for you.

- Tea. Most herbal teas (and especially Medicinal Strength Teas) involve the use of herbs that have anti-oxidant properties useful in prevention of cancer, heart disease, high blood pressure. Since these teas usually do not involve caffeine and other associated chemicals they are better from a health perspective than regular tea or coffee.

- Vitamin D. The human body (especially skin) develops its own vitamin D. It is necessary to maintain normal levels of calcium and phosphorous. A direct result of vitamin D deficiency is a weaker skeleton, a condition known as osteoporosis where the bones become porous and hence break easily. Vitamin D herbal supplements can help prevent osteoporosis.

- Selenium. This is a chemical so volatile that it does not occur in its free state in nature. Toxic in large amounts, trace amounts of it form the center of some enzymes that are vital to the normal working of all cells in nearly all living organisms. In the human body it behaves as an anti-oxidant and is also important for the normal working of the thyroid gland. Cereals, meat, fish, and eggs are good sources of selenium. Since the majority of sources are animal based, vegans and vegetarians should seriously herbal dietary supplements containing selenium.

- Vitamin A. This vitamin is responsible for maintaining good eye sight and promoting bone growth. It is also an antioxidant. Most skin and eye problems are related to vitamin A deficiency so if you have any such conditions, consider an herbal diet supplement rich in vitamin A.

Why Should You Try Herbal Diet Supplements?

Here is a crash course in the advantages of herbal supplements and medicines:

- They are cheap. Did you look at your medical bills for the past year? Now add up all that you paid the pharmacist for prescription and over-the-counter medications. Is the number looking scary yet? So if you have been using conventional medicine for small problems like common cold and stomachaches then perhaps it is time you considered herbal medicine. It might give you a healthier wallet or purse besides a healthy body.

- You can do it. Did you know that herbal medicine and supplements can be assembled in your own kitchen? There are thousands of herbal recipes available on the Internet. Just follow them like a recipe to bake a cake and there you are. Your medicine made by your own hand. If you have a garden you could even grow your own herbs.

- They are natural. Man has learned to do many things but nature continues to know more. So matter how much noise the pharmaceutical companies make you should at least give some time to listen to nature and her own remedies.

CHAPTER 7- THE SIDE EFFECTS OF GOING NATURAL

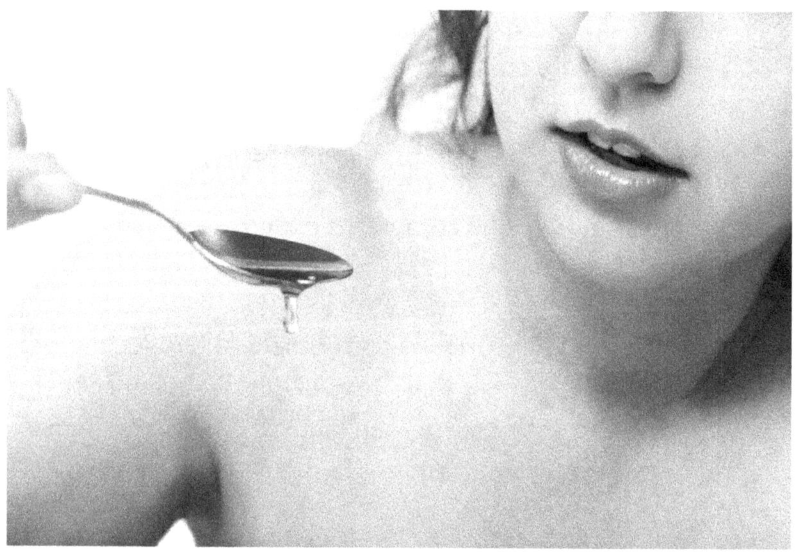

A scientific study has found that, though for the most part herbal supplements seem harmless, some of the more popular products pose a very special risk. This particular supplement interacts with and reduces the effectiveness of the drug saquinavir. The only thing to do for the moment is to avoid taking herbal supplements if you are being treated with saquinavir.

Herbal supplements are meant to boost our immune system, provide more ready energy, and improve general health. Though scientists say that research that is more extensive is required to determine which herbal supplements can have an adverse effect on our body, or, can interact with other medications and reduce their effectiveness, they remain united in their stand that several of the so-called harmless supplements can prove very harmful. Some of the more popular herbal supplements are chondroitin, ephedra, Echinacea, and glucosamine.

Chondroitin is typically used in the treatment of osteoarthritis. One side effect of chondroitin can be bleeding complications. This is more like when used in combination with a regular prescription drug that causes blood thinning.

Ephedra used to be a big favorite among people looking for a fat loss supplement. Ephedra promotes weight loss, provides energy boosts, and can also be used to treat respiratory tract problems like asthma and bronchitis. Recently, the FDA banned Ephedra because of dangerous side effects like high blood pressure, increased heart rate, false increase in metabolism, all which could lead to a cardiac arrest, heart arrhythmia, stroke, and might even be fatal in some cases.

Echinacea helps in the prevention and treatment of viral, bacterial, and fungal infections. It also helps in curing chronic wounds, ulcers, and arthritis. On the other hand it can cause immunosuppression that will cause the body to lose its self-healing capacity so wounds will not heal on their own. Immunosuppression also reduces the effectiveness of the immune system making infection easier.

Glucosamine is very often administered along with chondroitin. It contains chemicals that mimic the function of insulin and can cause the body to misbehave when this artificial insulin enters the blood stream. It can be especially bad for diabetics.

Other herbals supplements suspected of adverse side effects include gingko Biloba, goldenseal, milk thistle, ginseng, kava, and garlic. It is highly advisable to seek the consultation of your doctor before taking any supplements, herbal or otherwise. More than informing you about potential health risk the doctor can give valuable advice about food, nutrition, and supplements.

Ayurveda

Ayurvedic cures are based on ancient formulae that have been written down in the ancient Ayurvedic traditions. The success of an Ayurvedic cure depends on the quality of its ingredients. Looking to plants for healing powers is an old idea and was embraced by the early physicians in ancient India.

Ayurveda is an alternative herbal medicine therapy from India that believes heavy metals are therapeutic. The FDA considers heavy metals very dangerous for consumption and that is why Ayurvedic medicines are sold as supplements rather than medicines in America. Ayurveda is one of the oldest of traditional medicine that first established the routine of proper diagnosis and herbal cures for several diseases.

Natural Herbal Nutrition Supplements

People who opt for natural supplements or a whole food diet usually also wish to include whole food vitamins. Natural herb based supplements are usually lacking in certain vitamins that are only found in the animal kingdom so including a vitamin supplement is a wise decision. There are many companies making these vitamin supplements.

One reason to prefer whole good vitamins is that they are not manufactured in a factory; they are as close to the natural form as it is possible for a packed product to be. When you go shopping for whole food vitamins, pay close attention and make sure you do not purchase products that have preservatives or additives. Some people might also prefer their supplements in liquid form.

In case a healthcare professional recommends you take supplements then it is your duty to make certain that the product you purchase is 100% natural and contains no synthetic chemicals. It is common for whole food products to contain a combination of vitamins, minerals, and other essential nutrients. You are not likely to find a whole food product that contains just one specific vitamin or mineral.

Eating whole foods and taking natural whole food vitamins is a good idea because they help to maintain healthy cells. Due to environmental pollution there arc too many free radicals floating about that can easily cause cellular damage.

Whole foods in all shapes can help repair that damage. Another healthy option is to include as many raw diets as you possibly can. Nowadays, thanks to pesticides, preservatives, chemical treatments, and other processes that are inflicted on foodstuff to make them healthier typically kill off a considerable proportion of important vitamins and nutrients. When you finally get these to your kitchen, the raw food is already deficient in nourishment.

Cooking only makes matters worse by washing away even more vitamins and minerals. Eating a raw diet ensures that you get the maximum out of your food. A raw diet will make you feel healthier.

The New Trend?

Despite the increase in popularity that alternative medicine and herbal therapy are enjoying since the late 20th century there are opponents to the belief that these alternatives are better than conventional medicines.

The growing number of adherents to the alternative therapies and herbal remedies nicely balances this out. These people have made the choice to lead a completely drug free life. According to them, even the legally manufactured and sold products by pharmaceutical companies are unhealthy because of their synthetic chemical base.

This trend is getting more widespread because nowadays there are more and more celebrities and rich public figures who are adopting the drug free lifestyle. These prominent examples prefer the use of alternative remedies for even simple problems like headaches, pains, and cramps. They steadfastly refuse the use of conventional medications and would not casually take an Advil or Aspirin because of their firm belief in the inherent health benefits that come from a drug free lifestyle.

Since herbal cures and remedies have been around for several millennia, it should not be surprising that the list of ailments they can cure and the number of cures they offer is exhaustive. There are wide arrays of symptoms, diseases, mental problems, and some physical deformities (acne), or embarrassing conditions like bad breath that can be effectively cured or greatly improved through the use of herbal remedies. And, after all, why not? Don't you ever wonder where prescription drugs and medications come from?

Everything has to have its roots in nature. There are no alien supplied medications. Every drug available on the market today once used natural substances. This changed when chemical synthesis in a factory led to rapid drug production. This was good because more people could be treated quickly and it made some pharmaceutical companies very rich. It turned out to be bad because those same pharmaceutical companies now refuse to acknowledge their roots in nature or to try and give some respectability to their parent science. Also, note that the same product when it is in a natural state requires less processing by the body as compared to its manufactured equivalent.

Natural products also tend to leave behind fewer toxins in the body and are therefore better than artificial products. A little bit of skepticism is only natural when it comes to abandoning a lifetime of faith and dependence in pharmaceutical drugs. What should be considered is the ever-increasing number of people who are adopting the herbal and natural way of life and actually benefiting from its outcome.

The fact that there are some bad companies out there putting out unreliable natural and herbal products only increases the skepticism. The marketplace is so bad today that on an average for every good product that are at least two or three competing and thoroughly useless products. The good guys are being drowned out by the bad guys who only want to make a quick buck in a high selling market. In such a situation, the responsibility rests with you to properly research the product and the company that is manufacturing it.

Look for testimonials and reviews published on third party, neutral web sites. What sort of approvals does the product have? Are the ingredients checked for purity? What is the natural source for ingredients? What are the manufacturing standards that are being followed? How long has the company been in this business?

These are all legitimate questions and usually you should be able to call up the company on a provided telephone number to have all your queries answered. It does not matter what is the reason for your decision to take herbal supplements. It could be that you simply want an improvement in general health or you might be trying to combat some symptom that indicates the deficiency of some essential nutrient missing from your diet. What does matter is that you remember that when you go shopping for the supplement of your choice.

An incorrectly chosen herbal supplement will plunge you into the group of people who think that all this "natural" business is so much humbug. A well-chosen supplement on the other hand just might make you a convert and have you spreading the "natural" gospel to everyone you meet for the rest of your life.

CHAPTER 8- ACHIEVING THE PERFECT SKIN NATURALLY

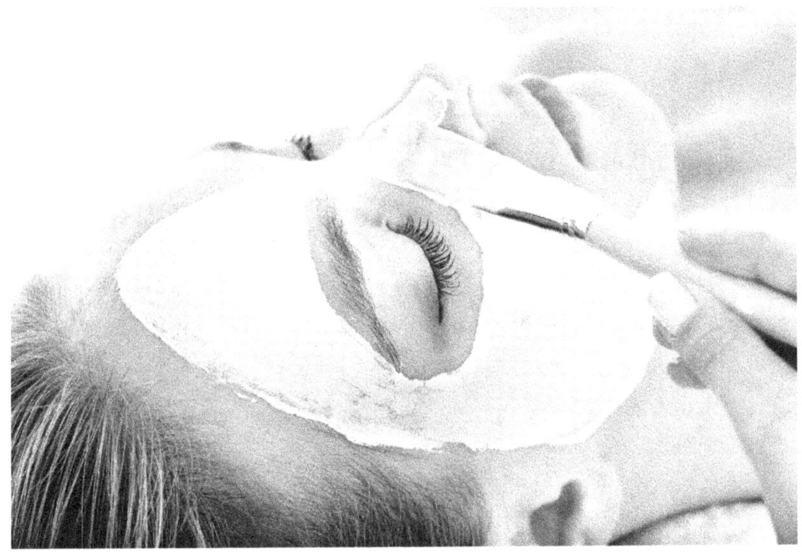

Organic skin care refers to the use of natural skin care products or therapies. The ingredients of these natural products are grown organically in places that are rich in nutrients, unlike similar products that are purely manufactured using synthetic processes and ingredients.

Organic skin care makes use of several different types of plants, extracts, herbs, flowers, and natural oils. Organic skin care products are merely an extension of natural skin care therapies. Organic skin care products are non-toxic and full of essential nutrients for the skin extracted from natural sources. These products nourish the skin and rejuvenate it gently.

Some of the problems they can cure are dark circles, wrinkles, and pimples. The overall effect of organic skin care products is younger and healthier looking skin. There are different organic skin care products available for the face and for other parts of the body.

Since the structure of skin is different depending on the part body it is important to choose the appropriate product. Apart from rejuvenating the skin, organic skin care products also have a soothing and healing effect on the body.

Some of the ingredients are quite rich in soothing essences that have a calming effect. Organic skin care products can make you feel fresh in addition to nourishing your skin. Newer products do not merely rely on plants and flowers. Some of them have already started using the special qualities of herbs and herbal extracts. Aloe vera, lavender, jojoba, olive oil, and rosemary extract are now regular ingredients in many organic skin care products. Nourishment of the skin takes place through cleansing, moisturizing, and toning.

Regular use of organic skin care products will ensure that your skin has no blemishes, pimples, or allergies. These products also keep the skin soft and supple. Healthy skin will produce fewer wrinkles because of its firmness.

Fight Acne

One of the more powerful forms of acne remedies is herbal. For people who are averse to taking strong acne drugs this is a very good option. The only problem with herbal remedies is that they are very slow acting and the results can take up to a month to become visible. Even so, herbal acne home cures are a good side effort to whatever other treatments being used.

The reason why herbal acne remedies take time is that these remedies depend on the body's capacity to metabolize fats and carbohydrates. Herbal remedies cure acne by encouraging the elimination of acne through the lymphatic system. There is a class of herbs called "alternative herbs". These herbs are basically used for the purpose of cleansing body tissues. They are herbs that help the body with the detoxification process. However, they do not remove the toxins from the body through normal elimination pathways like lungs, kidneys, or colon.

While they are not so popular in western culture, herbal acne remedies have a long history of successfully treating acne problems and they are so harmless that you should at least give them one try. Moreover, since most herbal acne remedies work inside the body they do not interfere with conventional topical (applied externally) acne medications.

Alternative herbs are very mild acting so there is no discomfort in their use. However, since they are mild by nature they take a longer time and consistent use to show results. Despite this, the fact remains the results are better and longer lasting. What is more, these herbs usually have a beneficial effect on the rest of the body. They can even be used to treat chronic inflammatory conditions. Some of the alternative herbs include burdock, cleavers, red clover, figwort, poke root, Echinacea, and blue flag. Like most herbal remedies these herbal acne cures are also best when a combination of herbs is used.

One frequently used and very popular combination is Echinacea, burdock, blue flag, and yellow dock. Just mix and prepare an infusion using hot water. Drink a cup about three times daily. If you wish to improve the flavor then please do not add sugar, instead, use honey.

A second combination is dandelion, sarsaparilla, and burdock. Mix them up when they are dry herbs. Prepare an infusion as before and have 3 cups a day.

A third decent combination for acne is lavender, yarrow, and elder flowers. Besides these, herbal acne remedies are available for topical use. Take the oil from a tea tree and apply it to the acne-affected area. This oil can be a bit strong so if you have sensitive skin just dilute it with water.

Fresh cabbage juice makes another great topical herbal cure for acne. This is also a better choice for people with sensitive who cannot stand tea tree oil. Calendula and chamomile can be used to make a very effective anti-inflammatory skin wash. Just prepare an infusion with these two as before but instead of drinking it let it cool. Store it in the fridge. When required, dab it onto affected areas.

Minerals like potassium phosphate and magnesium phosphate are also good for the skin. Zinc aids in the prevention of scarring. Vitamin C helps in healing acne lesions as well as acting as an antioxidant. These are but a few cases of how herbal acne remedies can be of help.

Creating Your Own Herbal Recipes

It is very easy to make your own herbal medicines. In fact, since most herbal remedies are best consumed when they are at their freshest you even have the best of all choices: grown your own herbs and make your own fresh remedies. However, it is important to have a thorough knowledge of the process of making your own remedies or even homegrown fresh herbs will go to waste.

Always keep in mind that unlike modern medicines herbal remedies are not a one-day affair. They take time to show their full effect because they work more gradually.

Bonnie Smith

When preparing your own herbal remedies always use a non-metallic or enamel pot.

Infusions are mostly tea-like beverages that are made by combining fresh herbs and boiled water. The common method is steeping. Typical ratios are about 1/2 or one ounce of herbs to one pint of boiled water. The mixture should be allowed to steep for at least 10 minutes. After that, you should strain the infusion into a cup.

Cold extracts make use of cold water instead of boiling water. The advantage is that unlike boiling some of the more volatile ingredients in herbs are not wasted in the extraction process. To prepare cold extracts, double the amount of herbal material and let it sit in cold water for about 12 hours then strain the mixture before drinking.

Decoction is a method of preparation that focuses on extracting mineral salts rather than vitamins. You should boil 1/2 ounce of herbs with one cup of water for 4-5 minutes. Steep the mixture for a couple of minutes before using it. Juice from herbs should not be made in a blender. Just chop and crush the herbs to squeeze out the juice. Add some water to this concentrate and then squeeze some more, drink it immediately. Do not store juice extracted this way.

Powder can be made from grinding your herbs when they are dried. The powder can then be taken with water, milk, or soup.

Ointments can be prepared by adding olive oil to a previously prepared decoction and then putting it on simmer until the water has evaporated. Beeswax may be included to improve consistency.

Essence can be prepared by dissolving one ounce of essential herbal oil in a pint of alcohol.

Chapter 9 - Using Aromatherapy

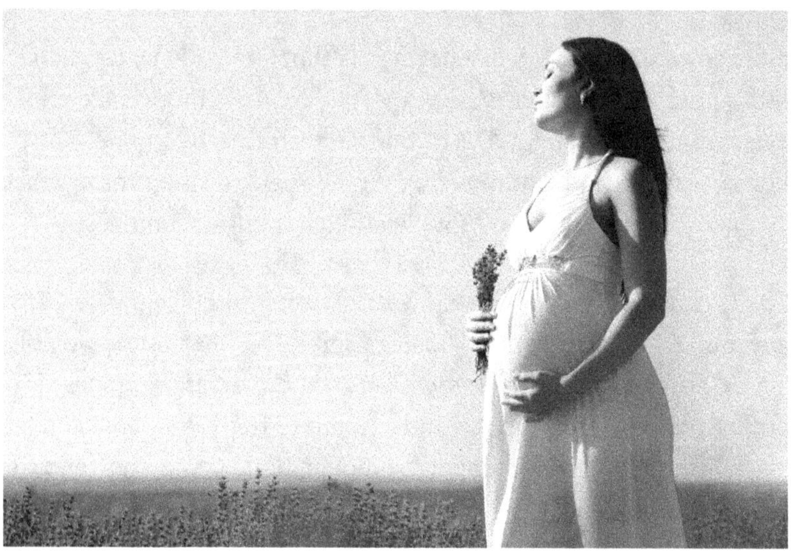

Aromatherapy uses herbal oils to treat the mental, emotional and physical properties of an illness through the sense of smell. Herbs are fragrant and give off particular scents that each have properties thought to help heal certain illnesses. Aromatherapy is thought to be especially helpful to calm nerves and soothe anxiety. Aromatherapy was used in prehistoric times, and has been used throughout history ever since. Incense is a form of aromatherapy that has been popular for centuries in many cultures.

Today, the use of aromatherapy is popular to help promote health and well-being and to reduce the effects of stress. Aromatherapy works by releasing herb infused oils or liquids into the air.

Essential oils may be placed onto a small cloth and then placed where the aroma can disperse throughout the area. Aromatherapy has become a popular and accepted method in the last several decades, and products are now widely available at local stores and supermarkets. Aromatherapy is used in many bath products and lotions. Examples of aromatherapy products include air fresheners or diffusers, as well as electric and battery powered products that spread the scent through the use of small fans.

Aromatherapy is a holistic approach to healing, taking into consideration the needs of the whole person. This takes into consideration your physical, mental and emotional states to help determine which essential oils are best suited for your particular situation. Aromatherapists mix essential oils together to create blends that are specific to your needs. Your sense of smell is the only sense that actually has nerve receptors exposed outside the body.

When a scent is detected special messages are transported to the limbic system inside the brain to be processed. The scent is identified there. This part of the brain also stores memories, which is why certain smells are often strongly associated with certain memories in your life. Blending essential oils together can form scents that are pleasant and relaxing, thus helping to reduce and eliminate stress and tension.

Essential oils are usually dissolved in either a water or oil base to blend together. The amounts used are small and do not cause any potential danger in these extremely low doses. These blends are often available as pre-made mixtures and are also able to be custom blended by an aromatherapist or by you at home. Massage therapy uses aromatherapy to help in relaxation.

Essential oils are used to massage the body. Besides the scent of the massage oil, small amounts of essential oils can also enter the body through the skin into the bloodstream. Again, these small doses are not considered harmful. Although aromatherapy does not claim to cure any diseases, it is, nonetheless, responsible for helping soothe the body and mind in many ways. It can help improve your mood and general feelings of well-being. Specific combinations of essential oils can help create euphoric sensations in the brain.

Aromatherapy can improve blood circulation and also improve lymphatic function when combined with massage therapy. Some soothing herbs are now used in common baby products to calm and help lessen the effects of colic and to help promote better sleep. Many herbs are used, and here are some of the most common herbs that are used in essential oils for aromatherapy.

Lavender - Lavender helps relieve tired muscles and can actually reduce muscle spasms. It is a very safe herb and is often used in many items, especially in baby products because of its gentle nature. There are relatively no side effects from using lavender. It is often used to calm anxiety and helps in eliminating insomnia. A diluted version is often used in a spray that can be used on beds and pillows to promote sleep. It is often used in small pillows that can be heated in the microwave and then applied onto the neck and back muscles to help relax them. Lavender blends well with most other herbs, making it a perfect choice for many herbal mixtures.

Bergamot - Bergamot is very uplifting. It is often used to help depression or mood swings. It is also helpful in eliminating insomnia and is said to help stop nightmares from occurring. It is a mild herb and is unlikely to cause any ill effects. It mixes well with most other herbs, including lavender, cedar wood, rosemary, geranium and lemongrass.

Tea Tree - Tea tree oil is an herb that is often used in topical mixtures to help fight bacterial infections. Used in aromatherapy, tea tree is said to help promote energy and helps relieve anxiety. It is also used to help aid in poor concentration. Another mild herb, tea tree is not associated with any known side effects and is safe to use. It mixes well with eucalyptus, bergamot, lavender and peppermint.

Neroli - Neroli is often used to help control the signs of stress and anxiety. Long used as a remedy, neroli is known to help those with exhaustion feel better and more relaxed. It helps with panic disorders and is said to calm fears, insomnia, and moodiness. It was used for many years as a treatment for grieving widows as it helps calm and soothe the mind. Neroli is a mild and safe treatment, and it blends well with most other herbs, including ylang-ylang, jasmine, Melissa and peppermint.

Melissa - Melissa is known for its antiseptic properties when used on the skin. In aromatherapy, Melissa is known to ease panic attacks. It is also used to help those who are overcoming addictions with alcohol or tobacco, as it helps alleviate those cravings. Melissa helps encourage calmness and brings serenity to you, and helps stop fear and depression. It mixes well with most other herbs, especially jasmine, neroli, geranium, and chamomile. Melissa in aromatherapy is mild, but when used on the skin it can cause irritation for those with sensitive skin. Test a small spot on the skin prior to use.

Frankincense - Frankincense has been used for thousands of years and has strong religious associations to the Bible. It is a popular herb used to help restore confidence and calm. It helps calm fears and paranoia, as well as nightmares. It helps restore balance to those who have signs of emotional exhaustion. It is mild and is unlikely to cause any adverse reactions, and mixes well with most other herbs, including ylang-ylang, myrrh, neroli, Melissa, cedar wood, rosemary and lavender.

Juniper - Juniper is commonly grown in the United States as well as Europe. The berries are very pungent and are used in the making of gin. Juniper is used to clear and stimulate the mind, and is said to prevent worry and unpleasant memories. It can renew enthusiasm and give you a new zest for life. It is safe as an aromatic; however, you should use caution when ingesting it if you have any kidney disease. Juniper blends well with most other herbs such as lavender, frankincense, tea tree and jasmine.

Herbs can be used in aromatherapy treatments in several ways. Essential oils are the easiest to use. These are made by distilling the plant material and mixing with a small amount of liquid or oil. Essential oils are concentrated and need to be diluted when used, and a few drops are all that is necessary when mixing with other oils. Essential oils can be used in baths, in lotions and perfumes and as inhalations. They are readily available at most health food or natural stores, as well as online. Do not put essential oils directly on the skin without first diluting them. These concentrations are strong and even safe herbs can cause irritations if not diluted. Be sure to dilute even more when using with young children.

Chapter 10 - Common Ailments and Their Natural Treatments

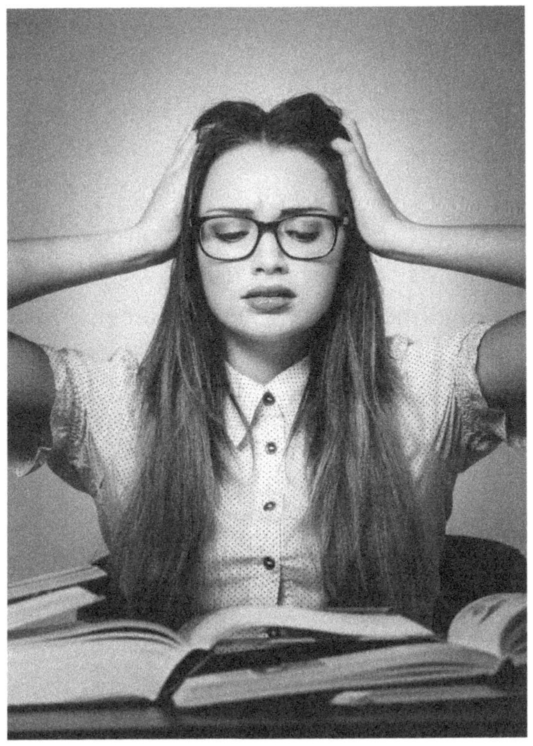

Altitude Sickness

If you are unaccustomed to higher altitudes, you may have feelings of sickness. These symptoms can range from mild to severe and may feel like a cold or flu. You may get a headache, nausea, weakness and may have trouble sleeping.

A headache is the most common complaint associated with altitude sickness. At higher altitudes the amount of oxygen mixed into the air is less. This drop of oxygen can affect the heart, muscles, lungs and nervous system. It can affect anyone, even those in good physical condition. After one to five days the body will begin to adjust and altitude sickness will subside.

Do-It-Yourself Herbal Treatments

The best way to avoid altitude sickness is to ascend slowly. You should also drink plenty of water and avoid drinking alcohol, because this can add to your symptoms. There are some herbs you can take to help prevent altitude sickness as well as lessen the effects on your body.

Begin taking these herbs from one to three days before you leave for the higher altitude.

- Ginkgo - Ginkgo helps improve circulation and therefore helps improve the body's tolerance to low levels of oxygen. Scientific studies have confirmed these results in humans. Take 120 to 150 milligrams daily. These are usually in the form of capsules. Although not common, side effects are possible. These include headaches and upset stomach.

- Reishi - This is an ancient Chinese remedy that helps to improve oxygenation to the blood. Take up to 1,000 milligrams in capsule form each day or two teaspoons of tincture three times per day. Herbalists suggest you take the dosage while at a higher elevation and continue taking it for several days after.

- Ginseng - Ginseng has been shown to help improve blood oxygenation and respiratory function. It is also used in treating asthma and bronchitis. Take up to four 500-milligram capsules daily while symptoms persist. Do not combine ginseng with caffeine, antidepressants or blood thinners, and do not use if you are pregnant or have high blood pressure.

- Siberian Ginseng - Well known as a tonic herb, Siberian ginseng helps improve overall health when taken long-term. Begin taking a few days before ascending for maximum effect. Take up to nine 500 milligram capsules per day or up to 20 drops of tincture up to three times per day.

- Ginger - Ginger is an old cure used for nausea. It can be used for altitude sickness as well as motion sickness. It comes in various forms such as tea, tincture, capsules or raw. Take up to eight 500 milligram capsules daily or ½ to 1 teaspoon of ground root per day or 10 to 20 drops of tincture per day. Dilute tincture in water to drink. Do not take ginger if you have gallbladder disease.

Anxiety

Anxiety is extreme stress, sometimes panic. It can cause symptoms such as shortness of breath along with feelings of doom. You can experience anxiety when your body reacts to signals it thinks are threats. Your heart rate goes up and you start to sweat. Other causes of anxiety can be classified as phobias, such as fear of flying or fear of heights.

Herbs can be an easy way to help ease anxiety naturally. If you are taking anti-depressant drugs, however, do not try to substitute herbal remedies. Talk to your doctor before taking herbal remedies. When treating anxiety, start with the mildest remedy in the mildest dosage and go from there. Many of the herbs used to treat anxiety are safely compatible.

- Oats - Oat seeds are calming and soothing and are helpful for those suffering from daily stress or who feels frayed. Tea is the common method of taking oats. Pour 1 to 2 tablespoons of seeds in a cup of hot water for ten minutes. You can drink a cup of tea every two hours as needed. Tincture is also available and you can take up to 3 teaspoons every two hours. Oats are also available as capsules.

- Chamomile - Used often as tea, chamomile has a very soothing and calming effect on you. It helps relax the muscles and also helps ease a tense stomach. Drink one cup of tea every two hours or up to 3 teaspoons of tincture every two hours. Chamomile is readily available as tea at most supermarkets, but it's a good idea to keep some on hand.

- Linden - Linden gently relaxes and eases muscle tension, and is also used as a remedy for high blood pressure. Linden also makes a good all-around remedy for helping keep the cardiovascular system functioning well. It is most often used in tea, and you should drink one cup of tea every two hours as needed. Tincture is also available as well as capsules.

- Vervain - Vervain is an herb that soothes and calms the nervous system as well as helps with depression. Often found as a tea, drink one cup of tea every two hours. It is also available as a tincture and in capsules.

- Motherwort - This old-time remedy is useful for the cardiovascular system in general. It can help calm nerves and aids in soothing anxiety that can cause a rapid heart rate. Drink one cup of Motherwort tea every two hours. It is also available as a tincture and as capsules. Consult your doctor before taking Motherwort if you are currently taking any cardiac drugs.

- Lavender - Lavender is relaxing and uplifting. It is fragrant and offers relief for anxiety and depression. Lavender essential oil is used diluted in bath water or can be inhaled. To use in a bath, add 10 to 12 drops to a full tub. You can also dilute it with oil to use as massage oil. It should not be taken internally.

- St. John's Wort - Commonly used to treat depression, St. John's Wort is an overall health booster that helps the nervous system. As a tonic, take up to 3 teaspoons every two hours. It is also available in capsule form.

- Skullcap - Used for anxiety and hormonal mood swings, skullcap is relaxing to the nervous system. It can be taken as a tea, a tincture or in capsule form. To make tea, mix one or two teaspoons of dried herbs in a cup of hot water for 10 minutes. Drink one cup of hot tea every two hours as needed.

- Kava-Kava - This is an anti-anxiety herb that originated in the South Pacific islands. It works similarly to Valium, working with the part of the brain that controls the nervous system and emotions. It does not cause addiction nor does the body build up a tolerance to it. It also doesn't impair thinking the way drugs may. In fact, in studies it was shown to improve brain function and memory. It is a good solution to treat anxiety on a short-term basis. The standard form is in capsules. Do not take with alcohol.

- Valerian - Valerian is considered a strong anti-anxiety herb. Similar to Valium, it works with the central nervous system; however it does not cause dependence. It is also used to improve sleep as well as a muscle relaxant. It is taken in capsule form. Note – a small percentage of users indicate an increase in anxiety when taking this herb. If that happens, discontinue use.

- Passionflower - Passionflower is a strong herb used primarily for calming and treating insomnia. It can also be used to help calm daytime anxiety. It is most commonly used as a tea. To make the tea, steep one to two teaspoons of dried herbs in a cup of hot water for 10 minutes. Drink one cup every two hours.

- Siberian Ginseng - This herb helps restore adrenal glands that are overstressed. It is a good choice for those who are chronically overstressed, and is taken as a tonic. It has a cumulative effect, meaning that it may take several weeks or even months to see results from taking the tonic.

Arthritis

Arthritis affects more than 40 million Americans of all ages. It is the stiffening or inflammation of the joints, and can occur in any joint, but it commonly starts in the hips, fingers and knees. There are two main types of arthritis, with osteoarthritis being the most common form. It is simply the breaking down or wearing down of the joints with age and worsens over time.

Rheumatoid arthritis is a form of an autoimmune disease that causes inflammation and distortion of the joints. There is no cure for arthritis, and doctors prescribe medication to help keep inflammation and pain down. Herbal remedies include both internal and external mixtures.

- Cayenne - Cayenne and other peppers contain analgesics and anti-inflammatory agents called capsaicin. This is often used in creams and other topical mixtures to help relieve pain. Creams come in different strengths.

- Evening Primrose - Taken internally, Evening Primrose helps combat inflammation. It can also help with the pain associated in particular with rheumatoid arthritis. Taken in capsule form, take up to 12 capsules per day. It can also be taken as oil, and you should take only ½ teaspoon of oil per day. Be aware that this oil can be expensive.

- Green Tea - Green tea has compounds that help the symptoms of rheumatoid arthritis. You'll find green tea products widely available now, and you may drink several cups of green tea per day, and black tea is also beneficial

- Yucca - Native Americans have used Yucca for centuries as food and as a remedy, and recent studies have confirmed its effectiveness as a remedy for arthritis. Yucca reduces the swelling and pain of arthritis as well as helps prevent stiffness in the joints. It can be applied topically to affected joints, and can also be taken internally. Capsules are available and you may take up to four 490-milligram capsules per day.

- Turmeric - Turmeric is a common Indian spice that is helpful in the treatment of arthritis, because it has anti-inflammatory properties. It can be ingested as well as used topically on affected areas. You can take 250 - 300 milligram capsules up to three times per day or up to one teaspoon per day in food. It is also available as a tincture.

Asthma

Asthma affects about 14 million Americans, many of them children. Asthma is a respiratory disorder triggered by certain allergens, and asthma attacks can come on suddenly and become very severe quickly. People with Asthma need to work closely with their doctor to find suitable remedies. The herbal remedies suggested here have been shown to help.

- Ginkgo - This ancient Chinese herb has long been used to help treat asthma, and studies have shown this to be particularly effective against exercise-induced asthma. Treatments require continued use for six to eight weeks at a time for maximum effectiveness. There have been rare cases of skin rash and upset stomach associated with the use of ginkgo. Check with your doctor if you are taking any blood thinners.

- Garlic and Onion - Garlic and onion have long been used to treat bronchitis and asthma, and they have been shown to inhibit allergen induced responses. The ingredient that possesses these characteristics is called Quercetin. It can be found as a dietary supplement in health food stores. Allicin, the ingredient in garlic, is available in capsule form as well.

- Licorice - This herb has anti-inflammatory properties as well as expectorant and anti-viral properties. It also has been known to stimulate the immune system, a huge factor in the treatment of asthma. Use products from the whole root, rather than the DGL form, which does not contain the active ingredient glycyrrhizin, which is necessary to get the effects desired. Do not take for longer than 6 weeks at a time. Also, do not take if you are pregnant, have high blood pressure or diabetes.

- Turmeric - Turmeric is one of the main spices in curry. It contains curcumin, which is known to work as an anti-inflammatory, anti-viral and anti-oxidant. You can easily add turmeric to your spice rack and use it when cooking. It is also available in capsule form and as a tincture. Do not take if you have gallstones.

- Ephedra - Ephedra has been known to help with asthma, however, it is no longer a recommended remedy due to possible side effects. Consult with your doctor before taking this herbal remedy.

Bladder Infections

Nearly half of all women suffer from a bladder infection at some time in their life. They are most common in sexually active and pregnant women. Bladder infections can become serious, so if it persists you need to see a doctor as the infection can travel to the kidneys where it can cause more serious damage.

- Cranberry - Yes, the old wives tale is actually true. Cranberry juice can help prevent and cure bladed infections by acidifying the urine. In order to be effective, though, you need to drink at least

5 cups of cranberry juice per day. You can also get cranberry in capsule form, which is easier to take. To prevent infections, drink 1-½ cups of unsweetened cranberry juice per day.

- Goldenrod - This herb is popular in Europe for treating bladder infections. It is one of the safest and most effective herbs for increasing urine flow and inhibiting bacteria growth. It also helps decrease inflammation. Taken as a tea, drink 2 to 3 cups of tea daily.

- Oregon Graperoot - The active ingredient berberine can help kill many types of bacteria that are harmful. It also helps prevent bacteria from sticking to the bladder wall, thus preventing bladder infections. Available as a tincture, take one teaspoon three times per day as needed. Do not use if you are pregnant.

- Echinacea - This acts as an anti-bacterial as well as an anti-inflammatory. It also is known to help pump up the immune system, which helps those with frequent bladder infections. If you have an allergy to ragweed, do not take this herb, as you could experience an allergic reaction.

Bronchitis

Bronchitis is an inflammation in the bronchi, the passageways from the lungs. It is characterized by a cough that starts dry and progresses to a mucus cough. Bronchitis can be acute or chronic. Acute bronchitis is usually the result of a cold and viral infection. Chronic bronchitis is a persistent cough that lasts more than 3 months, with air pollution and smoking contributing to chronic bronchitis. Herbal remedies can help with both types. If you are having severe symptoms such as chest pain, high fever or are coughing up blood you need to see a medical specialist immediately.

- Licorice - Licorice soothes mucous membranes and is an expectorant. It also helps stimulate the cells to produce more interferon, the body's own antivirus. Taken as capsules or as a tincture or tea, licorice should not be taken for longer than 6 weeks.

- Horehound - Horehound is available in syrups and also in lozenges. It soothes a sore throat and also works as an expectorant. It is also commonly available as a tea.

- Peppermint - Peppermint has menthol properties that help relax airways and also helps fight viruses. It is a good thing to use as an herbal steam. Add 3 to 5 drops of peppermint essential oil to 4 cups of very hot water. Then use a towel to cover your head and tent the steam. Inhale this way until the water stops steaming.

- Mullein - A tea or tincture, mullein is used to help you expel mucus. It can also help stop the pain of a raspy cough. Drink up to 6 cups of tea per day.

- Wild Cherry Bark - Wild cherry bark is often mixed with other herbs. It helps to suppress coughs, and should only be used for short periods of time. It is best used on coughs that are the dry, hacking type. It is available in teas and tinctures.

Burns

Burns of many kinds are common, and occur to all age groups. They can range from minor to major and are given categories based on severity. First-degree burns affect only the outmost layers of skin. Second-degree burns extend deeper into the skin and produce more redness and swelling as well as blisters. Third-degree burns are the most severe and often require skin grafts. First and second-degree burns can be treated quite easily with topical herbal remedies. Always see a doctor for severe burns or burns that cover areas of your body larger than your hand.

- Aloe - Aloe is a common burn aid and is found in many over the counter products. It not only helps soothe the pain but also fights bacteria and reduces inflammation. Find aloe in the gel form if possible and look for products that contain 100% aloe, as they work the best. If you have an aloe plant you can actually use that as well. Cut a piece off one of the "arms" and place the gel-like inner substance right onto the burn area. Aloe works well on sunburns as well as other minor burns.

- Calendula - Calendula helps as an anti-inflammatory as well as an antiseptic, and helps in the healing process. Calendula can be found in many over the counter products. For use on burns, find a product that is not too thick. You want the skin to be able to breathe through it.

- Comfrey - The active ingredient allantoin helps tremendously in speeding up the healing process of burns. Commercial products are available but you can also use a tea-soaked cloth placed on the burn. To use tea, first steep the tea in hot water for 10 minutes and allow cooling. Then, soak a clean cloth or towel in the mixture and apply to the burned area for a half-hour at a time.

- Gotu Kola - A compound in gotu kola helps to stimulate collagen growth to help repair skin. It helps heal burns and all types of wounds and helps keep scarring to a minimum. Apply topically by mixing the powder from capsules with aloe and then applying to the burn area.

Canker Sores

Also known as mouth ulcers, these sores can be painful. They are often associated with food allergies, immune system dysfunction and nutritional deficiencies. If you have them often, talk to your doctor to help determine the cause. Vitamin B12 and folic acid deficiencies can contribute to the cause of canker sores.

- Chamomile - a study has shown that chamomile mouthwash is an effective treatment for mouth sores. It helps keep inflammation down and helps promote healing. Drink up to 4 cups of tea per day or cool and use as a mouthwash. You can also make a mouthwash using 10 drops of tincture mixed with water.

- Echinacea - Echinacea tincture produces a numbing effect that is helpful in managing the pain associated with canker sores. If the canker sore is large or deep avoid using tinctures as they may cause stinging. Instead, use less concentrated mixtures such as tea.

- Gotu Kola - Gotu Kola is used to help promote healing. It has long been known to speed the healing of wounds. It can be taken internally as a hot tea or cold as an oral rinse.

- Goldenseal - Goldenseal has antiseptic and anti-inflammatory properties and can help to fight the infection associated with a canker sore. It also can help lessen the pain. Dissolve several drops of tincture in a glass of water and use as a mouth rinse.

- Ginkgo - When applied topically, this herb helps promote healing. It is rich in anti-oxidants and is also an anti-inflammatory. Make a tea and use the mixture to swab the sore with a cotton swab.

Bonnie Smith
Cold Sores

Cold sores are small blisters on the lips caused by the herpes simplex virus. They are often brought on by stress, and can last up to 14 days. While oral antiviral drugs may be prescribed by your doctor to lessen the effects, these have side effects of nausea and headaches. Repeated use of anti-viral drugs can cause viral resistance.

- Lemon Balm - Lemon balm is an herb that helps to stop the spread of many viruses, including the herpes simplex virus. Lemon balm is often found as an ingredient in commercial creams. Apply to the affected area up to five times per day as needed. It is also available in capsule form and as a tea to be taken internally.

- Licorice - Licorice is a natural anti-inflammatory and in studies has been shown to inactivate the herpes simplex virus. You can apply a licorice compress topically as often as needed. You may also take licorice internally in the form of tea or capsules. Do not use longer than 6 weeks at a time, and do not take if you have heart disease or high blood pressure.

- Mullein - The healing properties of this plant helps fight the herpes viruses, and can also soothe irritated skin. You can take it internally, as a tea, or apply topically in a compress.

- St.-John's-Wort - St.-John's-Wort contains the compound hypericin, which is known to help fight the herpes virus as well as to help heal wounds. Take 300-milligrams up to three times per day in capsule form. You can also drink tea made from steeping the dried herb. It can also be applied topically by making into a compress. Do not take internally if you are already taking a prescription anti-depressant.

Colds or the Flu

Colds and flu are often viral infections for which there is no cure. There are no drugs that can be taken as a preventative measure against the common cold. While there are many over the counter drugs available to treat the symptoms of colds and flu, you are often just as well off taking herbal remedies, which have fewer side effects.

- Echinacea - Studies have shown that this herb can shorten the duration and lessen the severity of a cold. It does this by helping to stimulate the body's own production of anti-viral substances and helps enhance the body's immune cells, helping it better fight off cold germs. Take 900 milligrams of Echinacea per day.

- Astragalus - This Chinese herb has immune-boosting properties, and also has anti-viral properties. Take Astragalus throughout the cold and flu season to help bolster your immune system to avoid getting colds. Commonly found in capsule form, take up to 3600 milligrams per day.

- Elderberry - Elderberry has been found to have compounds that help fight the flu. Take it as soon as symptoms start, and continue taking it daily. Commercially available as syrups and lozenges, these can be taken as directed on the package. It is also available as tea, tincture and in capsule form.

- Garlic - Garlic helps boost the immune system and fights bacteria and yeast. You can eat garlic in foods, but during cold season it is helpful to take a garlic supplement. It is readily available in capsule form. Take up to 5,000 micrograms per day.

- Vitamins - Vitamin C and Zinc are known to help lessen the duration of colds as well as help keep the symptoms down. Take supplements in capsule form or in lozenge form during cold season and especially with the onset of any symptoms.

Constipation

Constipation can happen to you when you have inadequate fluid or fiber intake. Laxatives are available over the counter. You can take an herbal laxative or use herbs to help your problem.

- Psyllium seed - These seeds help provide proper fiber in order to keep your system working properly. Available as a powder, it can be added to liquids. Dissolve a tablespoon in an 8-ounce glass of water or juice and drink immediately. Follow with another glass of water. This should be taken daily.

- Flaxseed - This is a bulking agent that provides a source of omega-3 essential fatty acids, something lacking in most diets. Mix one teaspoon of ground flaxseed in a glass of water or juice. You can take this up to three times per day.

Dandruff

Dandruff is an inflammation of the skin on the head, causing flaking and itching skin on the scalp. Often noticeable, it can be treated with herbal remedies to help keep the flaking to a minimum. Doctors are not sure what causes dandruff but it can flair up during stressful times as well as in the winter when the air is dry.

- Evening Primrose - Evening primrose contains oil that helps rashes as well as dandruff. You can rub the oil into the scalp to help keep the dry skin lubricated. You may also take it in capsule form, typically taking up to 10 capsules per day.

- Flaxseed - This has high levels of omega-3 fatty acids which have been known to help with rashes and dandruff. Usually taken internally, take 1 teaspoon per day. You can also rub flaxseed oil directly onto the scalp.

- Tea Tree - Known for its anti-fungal properties, tea tree oil is used externally. Add it to evening primrose oil or flaxseed oil and rub the mixture into the scalp before bed. Leave it on overnight, then rinse out in the morning and wash your hair as usual.

Depression

Everyone suffers from some depression from time to time. Depression is a hopeless, sad feeling that doesn't quickly go away. Depression may range from subtle to serious, and the more serious the depression, the more you need to seek medical help. If your depression is not severe, there are some herbal remedies that may help you. Do not take herbal cures while taking prescription medication and do not stop taking your medication unless directed to do so by your doctor.

- St.-John's-Wort - This herbal remedy is known for its use to treat depression. Studies have shown that the use of St.-John's-Wort is often as effective as prescription medications and has fewer side effects. You must take this for up to two weeks to start to see the benefits. Take it in capsule form and follow the directions for use or you can also take it as a tea. It can cause mild stomach upsets or rashes in some people.

- Kava-Kava - This herb helps alleviate anxiety that often accompanies depression. It can be taken without the usual side effects of prescription medication that makes people feel sedated. Taken in capsule form, take up to six 500-milligram capsules per day.

- Oats - This plant helps with depression and stress and helps with your overall nervous system. It is the same plant used to make the oatmeal breakfast cereal. Available as a tea, drink up to 3 cups of tea per day.

Diarrhea

Many things, such as virus or bacteria as well as food poisoning can cause diarrhea. Most diarrheas go away on its own in a matter of a few days. If it lasts longer than a week or is very severe you should see a doctor. There are some herbal remedies that can be very effective in helping treat it.

- Agrimony - Agrimony contains an astringent, which has drying properties in the bowel. Available as a tea, steep the dried herbs in hot water for 10 minutes. Then remove the herbs and drink the tea. You may drink up to 3 cups of tea per day as needed.

- Blackberry and Raspberry Leaf - Another astringent, the roots of these plants can help relieve diarrhea. Taken as a tea, you can take up to 3 cups of tea per day.

- Oregon Graperoot and Goldenseal - These related herbs contain berberine, which has been shown to be effective in treating the bacteria that can cause diarrhea. Available in capsule form, take up to 6 500- milligram capsules per day.

- Apples - Apples are a natural source of pectin, which is a very common anti-diarrhea remedy. Pectin is an ingredient in many over the counter remedies that helps add bulk. Eat apples or applesauce, but avoid apple juice as this tends to have the opposite effect.

Ear Infections

Ear infections are common in swimmers, thus a common name for one type of ear infection is "swimmer's ear". Ear infections are common in small children because their ear canals and tubes are not large enough to keep fluid from accumulating in them when they have a cold or flu. The accumulated mucus can become infected. Taking herbal cures instead of antibiotics can often help cure the infection. Besides taking herbs to help cure the infection, you can also try making some "swimmer's drops" to put into the ear.

- Echinacea - Taken internally, this ancient Chinese herb is known to help treat infections. You may take capsules or a tincture, and is also available as a tea. Note that you may be allergic to this herb if you are allergic to ragweed or other members of the aster family.

- Astragalus - Another ancient Chinese remedy that is taken orally, Astragalus is helpful in treating infections, and can be taken as a preventative remedy. Available as capsules or in tincture form, this is usually safe for children. For young children, check with the doctor before administering.

- Oregon Graperoot - The berberine in Oregon Graperoot acts as a natural antibiotic. It is used to kill many types of bacteria. It is taken internally in capsule form, and you should follow the directions on the bottle. Do not take if you are pregnant.

- Lemon Balm - A good-tasting herb, lemon balm is a natural anti-virus, bacteria fighting herb and is also used to help calm or soothe. Commonly available as a tea, drink up to 4 cups of tea per day.

Eczema

Eczema is a dry skin condition that affects many adults and children. It occurs in patches that can become thick and red, and it can often occur in those with allergies such as hay fever. Topical creams can be applied to help the skin recover. Herbal remedies do not have the side effects that some prescriptions can have.

- Licorice - The anti-inflammatory properties of licorice helps calm the skin when eczema flares up. It acts much like cortisol but without the side effects. It can be taken internally as a tea or externally by making a compress of the steeped herbs.

- Burdock - Known to decrease inflammation, burdock is a traditional herb, which has been used for years to help skin disorders. Besides helping inflammation, it also contains insulin that helps the body fight off skin bacteria. Drink up to 4 cups of tea per day. It can also be used topically. Simmer the dried root in hot water for 10 minutes. Strain and apply the cooled liquid to the affected skin area.

- Echinacea - Echinacea is American wildflowers that have substances that can help fight infection as well as decrease inflammation. It can be found as a main ingredient in many prepared herbal skin crèmes.

- Comfrey - Comfrey contains allantoin, an ingredient in many skin lotions. It soothes the skin and helps speed up healing. Apply as a salve or lotion. Do not use if pregnant.

Gas

Gas or flatulence occurs in everyone. If your gas is severe it can become uncomfortable and painful. Certain foods are known to produce gas, and you can avoid these foods if gas is a problem for you. These foods are broccoli, potatoes, dairy products and beans. Swallowing too much air while eating can also produce gas. There are some herbal remedies that can help treat gas.

- Peppermint - Peppermint contains menthol, which helps stimulate the intestines. It also helps relax the muscles in the digestive tract, promoting burping. You can eat peppermint candy or mints, which are helpful (Do you always notice the peppermint candies at restaurants?) Peppermint tea is also a great way to take peppermint. You can drink 1–2 cups of tea after a meal to aid digestion.

- Chamomile - Chamomile helps aid digestion and can also help dissipate gas in the body. It is also used as an anti-inflammatory. Often used as a tea, it is helpful to drink a cup of chamomile tea after eating. Those with allergies to ragweed should avoid this herb.

- Aniseed - The seeds from the anise plant have been shown to help eliminate gas buildup. Taken as a tea, pour the dried, crushed seeds in hot water for 10 minutes. Strain and drink warm.

- Ginger - Ginger root is known to help relieve nausea and helps with simple indigestion such as gas. You can drink a cup of tea after a meal that may cause gas. It is also available in capsule form.

Hay Fever and Allergies

Hay fever is an allergy to certain weeds and flowers that occurs most often in spring and summer. Allergies occur year-round. People can be allergic to many things, but the most common allergies are to pet dander and pollen. Herbal remedies are most effective for those with mild forms of allergies. If you are currently taking prescription medication for allergies consult your doctor before taking herbal remedies.

- Stinging Nettle - Studies have found that this herb works as well as conventional medications for treating the symptoms of hay fever. Stinging nettle is available in capsule form.

- Peppermint - The anti-inflammatory properties of peppermint help to calm mucous membranes. The scent of peppermint when inhaled helps you feel as though you can breathe easier. You may drink tea or you can steep the peppermint and breathe in the steam.

- Licorice Root - The anti-allergy properties of licorice act similarly to cortisone drugs but without the side effects. For hay fever, be sure to get whole licorice, not the type labeled DGL, which is used for ulcers.

- Garlic - Garlic contains an anti-inflammatory substance called Quercetin, which can help calm an allergic response in the body.

Headaches

Headaches occur in everyone from time to time. They are commonly a dull ache that happens in the temple or forehead and comes on during the day. Migraine headaches are a result of insufficient blood flow to the brain, and should be treated by a doctor to determine any underlying cause. Herbal remedies can be helpful in treating regular headaches, and be sure to drink water when you have a headache. Many low-grade headaches are actually caused by a mild form of dehydration.

- Feverfew - Feverfew contains substances that inhibit the release of mood hormones in the brain. For best results, use fresh feverfew. When that isn't available, take as a tea or in capsule form.

- Bay - There have been some doctors who recommend taking feverfew with bay to prevent a migraine headache. You can often find a combination available in a health food store.

- Ginger - Ginger has long been known to relieve and also to prevent headaches. It is an anti-inflammatory and also has substances that help reduce pain. Take in capsule form, according to directions.

- Peppermint - Taken internally or used externally, peppermint can help relieve a headache. To take internally, drink peppermint tea. To use externally, mix several drops of peppermint oil with lotion or body oil and massage into the temples.

Hemorrhoids

Hemorrhoids are painful swollen and inflamed tissues near the rectum, and they may burn and itch. Herbal remedies can actually help strengthen the blood vessels and reduce inflammation associated with hemorrhoids.

- Ginkgo - This helps strengthen the blood vessels and also has anti-inflammatory properties. Taken internally, it can be used as a tea, tincture or in capsule form.

- Horse Chestnut - This has long been used as an anti-inflammatory, as it helps to decrease swelling. It is also astringent, which helps lessen bleeding. You can use this herb topically in a cream or internally as a tea or in capsule form. To use externally you can use strong-brewed tea to soak the affected area.

- Witch Hazel - Witch hazel is a common remedy that is available at the drug store. Apply topically to the affected area, and do not take internally.

- Dandelion - Dandelion roots have laxative properties that help with constipation that often accompanies hemorrhoids. To make a tea, steep dried, chopped root for 10 minutes in hot water. Strain and drink warm.

Indigestion

Indigestion is common and happens to everyone at one time or another. Occasional indigestion can be easily treated with herbal remedies. If your indigestion is frequent or severe it could signal an underlying problem and should be checked out by a doctor.

- Chamomile - Well known as a soothing herb, chamomile tea can help dispel gas and relax tense stomach muscles. Taken as tea, drink 3 to 4 cups of hot tea per day. You can also use this as a tincture.

- Peppermint - Mint aids in digestion because it acts as a muscle relaxant in the stomach and can help calm the whole digestive tract. To be most effective use the tincture or essential oil mixed into water and drink. If heartburn is your problem, peppermint may aggravate the esophagus.

- Marshmallow - This plant is used to soothe the mucous membranes in the digestive tract. The root is the part of the plant that is typically used. Most often used in capsule form, take up to 6 500-milligram capsules per day.

- Angelica - Angelica stimulates digestion, calms nerves and can help dispel gas and bloating. It is often included in preparations with other herbs, such as dandelion. This herb may cause sensitivity to the sun.

Insect Bites and Stings

Insect bites are usually harmless but can be annoying and painful. They can cause pain and inflammation to the spot of the bite. Herbal remedies can be helpful in dealing with both the pain and swelling of the insect bite. If you are allergic to insect stings, are stung multiple times or are stung on the neck you should seek medical attention.

- Aloe - The soothing properties of aloe help hasten healing. It also has anti-bacterial properties. If you have a live plant simply cut a small piece of leaf and scoop out the gel and applies to the bite. Commercial aloe products are readily available at drug stores.

- Witch Hazel - Witch hazel has astringent properties and helps shrink swollen tissue. Apply to the bite with a clean cotton swab. It is a good idea to have this on hand for emergencies.

- Calendula - Calendula is an anti-inflammatory, anti-bacterial herb that helps wounds heal. It can be found in many commercial preparations at your local health store. Apply directly to the sting as needed.

- Comfrey - A substance called allantoin is found in comfrey, which has antiseptic properties and also promotes healing. You can use fresh, crushed comfrey leaves to apply directly to the bite. It is also available in many salves and lotions. Do not ingest.

Insomnia

Insomnia affects millions of people - there are times when you just can't get to sleep. Instead of taking prescription medications that can be harmful or addictive, try an herbal cure.

- Valerian - This herb is known to help you sleep and does not have any side effects, such as morning grogginess that is associated with prescription medications. It can help improve sleep quality as well. Take in capsule form according to package directions.

- Lemon Balm - Most often available as a good tasting tea, this herb not only helps ease insomnia but also calms nerves and fights fevers. It is also good for headaches and helps calm the digestive tract.

- Passionflower - This herb has been shown to calm nerves and decrease anxiety. If you suffer from sleeplessness due to an overactive mind, this will help calm it. Take as a tea before bedtime. Do not mix this herb with MAO antidepressants.

- Kava-Kava - This herb helps calm and relax muscles and is known to aid the brain in promoting sleep. Take in capsule form according to the instructions. Do not take kava-kava if you are taking sedatives, and do not use while pregnant.

- Chamomile - Chamomile is known for its relaxing properties, and is a gentle sleep aid. Most effective in tea form, drink a cup of warm chamomile tea before bed.

Irritable Bowel Syndrome

IBS is a very common ailment that particularly affects women, but can also affect men. The symptoms are constipation and diarrhea with severe bloating and cramping. If your IBS happens infrequently, try these herbal remedies.

- Peppermint - Peppermint is helpful in many digestive disorders because it has soothing properties in the digestive tract. It helps stop cramping and is an anti-inflammatory. Use peppermint oil in capsule form to be most effective in treating this problem.

- Psyllium - These seeds help aid the intestinal tract whether the problem is constipation or diarrhea. Stir the dried seed husks into a large glass of water or juice and drink immediately. Drink one glass per day to keep IBS at bay.

- Chamomile - Chamomile helps calm the stomach and intestinal tract. It helps to stop muscle spasms that sometimes occur with IBS. You can drink as a tea, up to 4 cups per day between meals. It is also commonly available in capsule form. Do not take if you have allergies to ragweed.

Menstrual Problems

Many women feel various symptoms that are associated with their menstrual cycle. These include moodiness, fatigue, cramps and headaches. While over-the- counter medications can help with some of the symptoms, you may want to try some herbal remedies that can help without side effects.

- Vitex - This tree berry extract is good for many menstrual symptoms, including fluid retention, moodiness, food cravings, and acne. It helps by regulating the pituitary gland. Take in capsule form. Do not use during pregnancy, and do not use if you are taking oral contraceptives, as vitex may lessen their effectiveness.

- Black Cohosh - Also used to help the symptoms associated with menopause, this powerful herb helps relieve cramps, and helps with pain as well. You must take this herb for a few weeks for it to be effective. Take 3 to 4 droppers of tincture twice a day.

- Cramp Bark - This herb gets its name from its use as an antispasmodic. It is safe to use and will relax uterine cramping. It can be combined with valerian or kava-kava. Take as a tea or in capsule form. You can find it mixed with other herbs in mixtures designed to treat PMS.

- Kava-Kava - A calming herb, kava-kava helps ease anxiety. It also has pain-relieving effects similar to aspirin. It is recommended to start taking this several days before your period and through your period.

Morning Sickness

Many pregnant women experience morning sickness during pregnancy. The exact cause is not known, however it is likely due to hormonal and metabolic changes that are occurring. Some herbs may offer help for morning sickness, but do not take any herbal remedy while pregnant until you discuss it first with your doctor.

- Ginger - Ginger helps calm the stomach and can stop nausea and vomiting. It is also a cure for motion sickness, and it can also reduce gas and bloating. The gentlest dosage is to take as a tea.

- Chamomile - Chamomile is soothing and gentle on the digestive system. It is best used as a tea to help calm and relieve nausea. You can sip the tea as needed throughout the day whenever you have symptoms of morning sickness.

- Peppermint - Soothing to the digestive tract, this gentle herb is safe to use. It can improve symptoms of bloating and gas. Steep a tea by putting 2 teaspoons of dried peppermint leaves into hot water for 10 minutes. Strain and drink the tea warm.

Nausea

Everyone has a bout of nausea from time to time. It can be brought on by the flu, but often there is no real reason for feeling nauseous. If you are sick, make sure you frequently drink small amounts of liquids to stay hydrated. Some herbal cures may help alleviate the symptoms.

- Ginger - Ginger is readily available in many forms and is safe to use. It is effective in reducing nausea and helps quiet the stomach. Extremely versatile, it can be taken as a tea, in crystallized form, dried, powdered or as a tincture. It is also available in capsule form.

- Peppermint - Peppermint settles the stomach, and you have probably noticed that peppermint candies are often given at restaurants. If you have a headache or a cold, peppermint is also a good choice for these ailments. Keep peppermint lozenges in the car to help tame nausea while driving. It can also be taken as a tea or tincture.

- Lemon Balm - Lemon balm helps the body to deal with and expel excess gas. It can also relieve spasms. The flavor is also pleasing. Make a tea by steeping dried herbs in hot water for 10 minutes, then strain and drink.

- Chamomile - This herb is useful for all sorts of ailments and acts to calm nausea. Mild enough for children, this herb is a safe choice in treating many illnesses. Use as a tea or put drops of the tincture into water and drink.

Pneumonia

Pneumonia often starts with a bad cold but spreads to the lungs, where it causes infection. You may have a mucous cough and may have difficulty taking a deep breath. Severe pneumonia often requires a hospital stay. Mild pneumonia may be treated with herbal remedies, especially if you are prone to this type of condition. Always have your condition checked by a doctor to ensure that it does not progress in severity.

- Echinacea - This immune boosting herb is often effective by helping the body fight off infections. This is available in capsule form as well as in a tea or tincture.

- Goldenseal - This herb helps fight bacteria and can also help stimulate the body's immune system. You can take this in capsule form or as a tea or tincture. In capsule form, take up to 1,000-milligrams three times per day.

- Mullein - This herb is known to help the respiratory tract and can help fight inflammation. It also eases coughs, helping the body get needed rest. Usually used as a tea, pour the dried root in hot water for 10 minutes. Remove the herbs and drink the tea. You may drink up to 3 cups of tea per day.

Sinus Infections

Sinus infections are infections of the sinus cavities, located in the cheeks, ears and forehead. Often caused by viruses, the infections can be particularly hard to get rid of. A bad cold or hay fever can turn into a sinus infection, and they often happen to people who smoke. They can sometimes effectively be treated with herbal remedies.

- Echinacea - This herb helps boost the immune system and is known to help fight off infections, particularly sinus infections. Take as soon as you feel an infection coming on and continue to take every two hours. You need to take it frequently at the onset of the illness in order to get the best results. You can take up to nine 400-milligram capsules per day.

- Astragalus - Taken over a long period of time, Astragalus helps boost the immune system slowly. It builds up the immune system of people who get sinus infections often, and is most commonly taken in capsule form.

- Oregon Graperoot - This herb is an antimicrobial, as well as astringent and an anti-inflammatory. It can be used to treat a number of infections, including sinus infections. Commonly found in tincture form, take 15 drops at a time up to three times per day.

- Garlic - Garlic has properties that help fight bacteria. Overcooking deactivates the ingredient that fights bacteria, so it is best used raw. Garlic capsules are widely available.

Smoking

Smoking is an addiction, which is difficult to stop once started. Many people want to quit smoking but have a hard time. People who quit smoking suffer through many withdrawal symptoms including nervousness, irritability and insomnia. Some herbal cures are available to help make quitting easier.

- Mullein - This herb helps soothe irritated lungs and mucous membranes in the respiratory tract. Take 2 to 3 cups of tea per day or ½ to 1 teaspoon of tincture three times per day.

- Coltsfoot - This herb helps soothe inflamed lung tissue and also helps to loosen secretions, making it easier to cough up. Drink up to 3 cups of tea per day. Take coltsfoot for no more than four weeks per year.

- Lobelia - This herb helps ease coughs and relaxes bronchial muscles. It also may help reduce nicotine cravings. Take as a mild tea, up to 3 cups daily. Lobelia has been known to cause nausea in some people so discontinue use if this happens.

Sore Throat

Many things can cause a sore throat, from postnasal drip, dry air, breathing through your mouth to a cold or virus. Antibiotics cannot treat viral infections, and left to run its course will last several days. Some herbs can soothe the symptoms of a sore throat and make it feel better.

- Echinacea - Echinacea helps boost the immune system and makes it function better, and has been known to kill some viruses of the respiratory system. It can be taken along with antibiotics to treat strep throat, as it will help speed recovery. Take in capsule form. Increase the dosage at the onset of illness and decrease after several days. Do not take if you have an allergy to ragweed.

- Licorice - The root of this herb helps reduce inflammation and stimulates the immune system, helping to fight infections. There are two types of licorice products. Be sure to find the licorice capsules that are for boosting the immune system and not the type used in treating ulcers.

- Eucalyptus - This is a fragrant herb that soothes a sore throat. It also has antiseptic properties and can help shrink swollen tissues. It is found readily available in throat lozenges, which are a convenient way to take it. You can also drink eucalyptus tea.

- Lemon Balm - Lemon balm is helpful in fighting off viruses and bacteria. Use as a tea - steep the dried leaves for 10 minutes in hot water. Strain and drink the tea warm. The tea can also be helpful when used as a gargle.

Sprains and Strained Muscles

Sprained or strained muscles may occur from overuse or exercise. Often, dehydration contributes to the sprain. Sometimes a long soak in a tub of hot water will do wonders to help replenish overused muscles. For regular sprains, apply cold packs for the first twenty-four hours after the injury. Also, keeping the injury elevated helps improve circulation and lessen the swelling. Some herbal remedies are also helpful for minor sprains and strains.

- Turmeric - Turmeric has been found to have strong anti-inflammatory properties and is helpful in treating many sports injuries, including sprains. It can be used topically but is most often taken internally. Take up to 1800 milligrams per day. Do not take more, because in larger quantities it can hurt the stomach.

- Kava-Kava - This herb is used to help relieve pain and as a muscle relaxant. Taken internally, you can take up to eight 500-milligram capsules per day. Do not combine kava-kava with alcohol or sedatives.

- Peppermint - The cooling sensation of the peppermint helps take away from the sensation of pain, helping to feel better. Use topically for a sprain. It is available as an ingredient in many commercial creams found at the health food store. You can also use peppermint oil added to massage oil to massage into the skin.

- Comfrey - Comfrey helps relieve pain, reduce swelling and inflammation. It is found in many over the counter salves and creams. It is effective without the side effects of many prescription medications. Apply as directed on the label.

Stress

Stress is unavoidable in our busy world. You can limit the amount of everyday stress you have by developing calming methods and through exercise. Some stress is dealt with through prescription medication. Herbal treatments can be very beneficial, but consult with your physician first if you are already taking medication.

- Siberian Ginseng – This herb helps boost the health of the adrenal glands, helping the body resist stress-related illnesses. It can also improve mental alertness. It is safe to be used as part of a daily regime. Take in capsule form following the directions.

- Panax Ginseng - This type of ginseng improves the body's ability to cope with stress. Used as a tonic, it is thought of as a fortification tonic. It is most often taken in capsule form. Herbal practitioners recommend using for two weeks at a time followed by a one-week rest before starting again. Do not take if you have high blood pressure, and do not combine with caffeine.

- Schisandra - Commonly used in traditional Chinese medicine, these berries can be used as a general tonic that helps counter stress and fatigue. It also helps increase mental function. Take up to six 580- milligram capsules per day.

- Kava-Kava - The root of this herb helps calm nerves without side effects associated with prescription medication. It is typically used in capsule form. Do not take with prescription drugs or alcohol, and do not drive while taking this herb as it acts like a sedative.

- St.-John's-Wort - A common treatment for anxiety and depression, it is also useful in treating the symptoms of stress. Studies have shown that it is as effective as Prozac and other anti-depressants. It is commonly taken as a tea and is also available in capsule form. Do not take with prescription anti-depressants unless instructed to do so by a doctor.

Toothaches

A toothache can bring sever pain. It signals a problem with a tooth or gum and needs to be looked at by a dentist. If you can't get to a dentist immediately, however, you can help ease the pain with an herbal remedy.

- Clove - Clove essential oil is a strong natural pain reliever. Used topically, buy clove essential oil at the health food store. Apply with a clean cloth or hold on the effected tooth with a cotton swab. Hold on for a few minutes, and it will gently numb the area.

- Turmeric - This spice is known as an anti-inflammatory and antibacterial, and it helps fight infection. You can mix the spice with water to form a paste and dab onto the tooth.

- Chamomile - Chamomile will help soothe the aching tooth and calm your nerves as well. It is known to fight infection and promotes healing. It is very safe to use. Drink as a tea or use the tea as a mouth rinse.

Ulcers

Ulcers are sores in the stomach or gastrointestinal tract, and they can be extremely painful. Get medical attention to determine the exact cause of the pain. Herbal treatments are useful for ulcers that are not severe.

- Licorice - Herbalists say that licorice works as well on ulcers as prescription medication, but without any side effects. It helps rid the body of harmful bacteria and induces healing. Look for the form of licorice called DGL, which is the best type to use on ulcers. It needs saliva to activate the helpful ingredients, so this herb is best taken as a tea or tincture. Your use should be limited to 6 weeks at a time unless instructed otherwise by a doctor.

- Chamomile - The calming properties of chamomile help heal the stomach and digestive tract. It decreases inflammation, and can also help calm nerves that perpetuate ulcers. Take as a tea or tincture up to 4 times per day.

- Calendula - Calendula helps promote healing and has astringent properties that can help stop bleeding. Take as a tea or tincture up to 4 times per day.

- Meadowsweet - This herb soothes the stomach and digestive tract. It reduces excess acid by soothing the stomach lining. It is available as a tea, and you should not use if you have an allergy to aspirin.

Warts

Warts are caused by a virus called the human papillomavirus, which has many strains. Common on the hands, they can pop up anywhere, especially on the face, feet and neck. You may want to try an herbal remedy to help remove warts. Remember that it can takes weeks to see any results from herbal use.

• Celandine - The sap from this member of the poppy family can help reduce or eliminate warts, and helps with other skin problems as well. If you have the plant, take some of the sap and dab it onto the wart daily. If not, you can brew some strong tea with the dried root and dab the mixture onto the wart daily.

• Black Birch Bark - The bark from the black birch contains antiviral compounds and salicylic acid, the same ingredients found in many over the counter wart removal salves. You can purchase the powder from a natural health store and make a paste by mixing some with water. Apply daily to the wart.

• Bloodroot - This herb is known to help heal warts and has been used for centuries. Get the powder form from a natural health food store, and mix with water to form a paste and apply to the wart daily.

• Dandelion - Some people claim the milk from a dandelion can remove warts. To try, simply pick the dandelion at the bottom and squeeze some of the milky inner substance onto the wart. Repeat daily.

ABOUT THE AUTHOR

Bonnie Smith is an aromatherapist. She runs a store selling essential oils and herbs. She is a notable authority in alternative medicine, particularly in aromatherapy.

Bonnie was born on June 12, 1960. She is the eldest of three sisters. Her parents were farmers so she spent her early years familiarizing the chores in a farm.

In college, Bonnie began to show an immense interest in scents and oils. She would often experiment on numerous ingredients to come up with a scent that would appeal to her and her friends. Her dorm mates would later note that whenever they step inside Bonnie's room, they are taken to another world – a realm of fragrant flowers and aromatic herbs.